PHILIP'S

GUIDE TO THE
HUMAN
BODY

RICHARD WALKER

D0269909

Essex County Council Libraries

EXECUTIVE ART EDITOR Mike Brown

DESIGNER Caroline Ohara

PRODUCTION Aggeliki Rabaouni

www.philips-maps.co.uk

First published in 2003 by Philip's,
a division of Octopus Publishing Group Ltd,
www.octopusbooks.co.uk
2–4 Heron Quays, London E14 4JP
An Hachette Livre UK Company
www.hachettelivre.co.uk

Second edition 2008

Copyright © 2003, 2008 Philip's

Text copyright © 2003, 2008 Richard Walker

ISBN 978-0-540-09004-4

Richard Walker has asserted his moral right under
the Copyright, Designs and Patents Act, 1988, to
be identified as the author of this work.

A CIP catalogue record for this book is available
from the British Library.

All rights reserved. Apart from any fair dealing for
the purpose of private study, research, criticism or
review, as permitted under the Copyright, Designs
and Patents Act, 1988, no part of this publication
may be reproduced, stored in a retrieval system,
or transmitted in any form or by any means,
electronic, electrical, chemical, mechanical,
optical, photocopying, recording, or otherwise,
without prior written permission. All enquiries
should be addressed to the Publishers.

Printed in China

FRONT COVER (CLOCKWISE):
left: Digestive system *(Philip's)*
top centre: Double helix of DNA *(Philip's)*
top right: Horizontal section through the eye *(Philip's)*
bottom right: X-ray of a female adult pelvis
                (Science Photo Library)

BACK COVER:
left: Skull *(Philip's)*
right: Electrical system of the heart *(Philip's)*

SPINE :
top: Horizontal section through the eye *(Philip's)*
centre: Cross section through the tooth *(Philip's)*
bottom: Double helix of DNA *(Philip's)*

PHOTOGRAPHY CREDITS

All photographs from Science Photo Library
8c L. Willatt, East Anglia Genetics
19bl James Stevenson
19br Dave Roberts
21br Mehau Kulyk
23tr Hugh Turvey
23bl Bo Veisland, MI&I
23br James Stevenson
24tr James Watney
25tl James Stevenson
25bl Bo Veisland, MI&I
25br Astrid & Hanns-Frieder Michler
33tr Don Fawcett
35br Prof. S. Cinti
38br Scott Camazine
41tr Francis Leroy, Biocosmos
43tl SPL
49tr Prof. P. Motta and Prof. T. Naguro
61 Russell Kightley
65 Francis Leroy, Biocosmos
69tr CNRI
72bl Biology Media
73t CNRI
73b CNRI
75 CNRI
109 Mike Bluestone
112 NIBSC
113 Alfred Pasieka
115 Alfred Pasieka
117 A.B Dowsett
120 Sidney Moulds
122 Barry Dowsett
123 CNRI
126 Alfred Pasieka
131 Simon Fraser, Royal Victoria Infirmary,
    Newcastle upon Tyne
132 SPL
135 Alfred Pasieka
137 John Bavosi
139 BSIP Ducloux / Brisou
142 John Bavosi
144 John Bavosi
145 Dr Andrejs Liepins
146 NIBSC
147 Lawrence Lawry
149 Dr Steve Patterson
150 John Bavosi
152 Claude Nuridsany & Marie Perennou
153 SPL
154 John Bavosi
156 NIBSC
157 Simon Fraser, Royal Victoria Infirmary,
    Newcastle upon Tyne
158 John Bavosi
161 Eye of Science
162 Dave Roberts
163 SPL
164 SPL
165 Sinclair Stammers
166 Alfred Pasieka
167 CDC
168 Wellcome Dept. of Cognitive Neurology
169 Sidney Moulds
170 Mehau Kulyk
171 BSIP VEM
172 Biophoto Associates
173 Dr Linda Stannard, UCT
174 Eye of Science
175 CNRI
176 Eye of Science
177 SPL
180 Sidney Moulds
181 CNRI
182 Scott Camazine
186 SPL
187 Eye of Science

Contents

THE STRUCTURE OF THE BODY

The human body is a living structure of incredible complexity. The purpose of this book is to describe simply yet comprehensively the anatomy (structure), physiology (function) and interdependence of the body's component parts. Throughout the book, for ease of description, specific terms are used to describe different regions of the body, and the orientation and position of body parts. This terminology, in common usage by doctors and scientists, is explained below.

Body regions

When viewed externally, the whole body is divided into regions, or areas. The **head** houses the brain and major sense organs. The brain is supported and protected by the skull, which also forms the framework of the face. The head is held upright by the muscles and bones of the neck, which connects the head to the trunk. The **trunk** (or torso) forms the central part of the body and has two sections. The **thorax** forms the upper part of the trunk and extends from the neck to the diaphragm. The **diaphragm** is a sheet of muscle that separates the thorax from the abdomen, the lower part of the trunk. The terms cephalic, cervical, thoracic and abdominal describe items found, respectively, in the head, neck, thorax and abdomen. The two upper **limbs** (or extremities) are each divided into three regions: the arm, forearm and hand. The hollow just beneath the junction between the upper extremity and trunk is the **axilla** (or armpit). The two lower limbs (or extremities) are each divided into the thigh, leg and foot. Most organs, such as the heart and stomach, are enclosed inside one of three closed cavities within the body. Females and males have the

Body regions

Neck

Thorax

Upper extremity

Trunk

Arm

Abdomen

Forearm

Penis

Scrotum

Thigh

Nipple

Breast

Vulva

same body regions, but their body shapes, and internal and external reproductive organs, differ.

Orientation and direction

The terminology that describes orientation and direction assumes that the body is upright, with arms at the side, and the palms of the hands facing forwards. Some terms refer to an imaginary midline, or axis, that runs vertically down the centre of the body and splits it in two.

- **Medial** means at or nearer to the midline, or on the inner side of; **lateral** means away from the midline, or on the outer side of. For example, the backbone is medial to the kidneys and the left eye is lateral to the bridge of the nose.
- **Superior** means above, or towards the head or upper part of the body; **inferior** means below, or towards the lower part of the body. For example, the superior

vena cava is a large vein that carries blood into the heart from the upper body and the inferior vena cava does the same from the lower body.

- **Anterior** (ventral) means towards the front of the body; **posterior** (dorsal) means towards the back of the body. For example, the heart is anterior to the backbone and the sacrum is posterior to the urinary bladder.
- **Proximal** refers to something that is nearer to the point of attachment of a body part; **distal** means farther away. The proximal end of a digit in the hand is at the knuckle, while its distal end is at the fingertip.
- **Superficial** is used to indicate something at or near the body's surface; **deep** means located away from the body's surface. For instance, the skin is superficial to the skeleton, while the brain is deep to the skull.

Body orientation

Body cavities

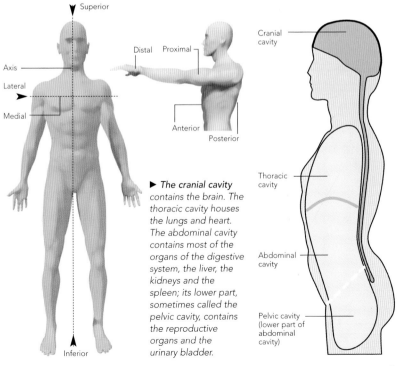

Superior

Distal   Proximal

Axis

Lateral

Medial

Anterior

Posterior

Inferior

Cranial cavity

Thoracic cavity

Abdominal cavity

Pelvic cavity (lower part of abdominal cavity)

▶ *The cranial cavity contains the brain. The thoracic cavity houses the lungs and heart. The abdominal cavity contains most of the organs of the digestive system, the liver, the kidneys and the spleen; its lower part, sometimes called the pelvic cavity, contains the reproductive organs and the urinary bladder.*

CELLS

Cells are the basic units of life. The body contains more than 100 trillion (100,000,000,000,000) cells that work together to form a functional human being. There are more than 200 different types of cells – including red blood cells, muscle fibres and nerve cells – each with their own particular role. All cells share the same basic structure. A thin, pliable plasma (or cell) membrane surrounds the jelly-like cytoplasm, which contains various organelles ('little organs'), such as mitochondria and ribosomes, each with their own function; the spherical nucleus is the control centre of the cell.

Plasma membrane

Merely 8 nanometres (0.000008 mm) in width, the plasma membrane forms a boundary that separates the cell from its surroundings and selectively controls what substances enter or leave the cell.

Many cell organelles, including mitochondria, are bound by a membrane or membranes with a structure similar to that of the plasma membrane.

Cytoplasm

The cytoplasm is the part of the cell that lies between the plasma membrane and the nucleus. It consists of a viscous fluid, the cytosol, which is 90% water and contains dissolved amino acids, salts, sugars and other substances and organelles. These include microfilaments (thin protein strands) and microtubules (hollow protein rods) that together form a cytoskeleton which gives the cell its shape and keeps other organelles in their correct positions.

Organelles

The organelles serve to divide the cytoplasm into separate, but linked, compart-

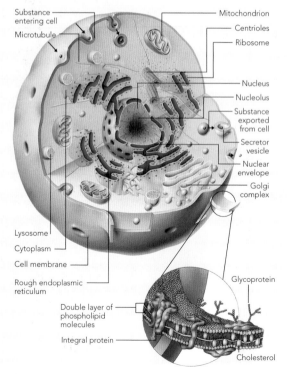

Labels (clockwise): Substance entering cell; Microtubule; Mitochondrion; Centrioles; Ribosome; Nucleus; Nucleolus; Substance exported from cell; Secretor vesicle; Nuclear envelope; Golgi complex; Glycoprotein; Cholesterol; Integral protein; Double layer of phospholipid molecules; Rough endoplasmic reticulum; Cell membrane; Cytoplasm; Lysosome

Cell and membrane structure This picture illustrates the organelles described in the text above. It also shows the detailed structure of the cell membrane. This consists of a bilayer (double layer) of phospholipid molecules that gives the plasma membrane its flexibility; simple substances, such as oxygen, pass through the bilayer by simple diffusion. It also contains cholesterol, another type of lipid, as well as proteins. Integral proteins pass across the membrane and act as channels to take substances into the cell by a process called active transport, which requires energy. Surface proteins – often attached to sugar molecules to form glycoproteins – act as 'flags' that identify the cell as 'self' to the body's immune system.

ments. This ensures that the many chemical reactions going on inside the cell do not interfere with each other.

• **Mitochondria** (sing. mitochondrion) are sausage-shaped organelles that act as the powerhouses of the cell. Using an oxygen-requiring process, called aerobic respiration, they release energy in the form of ATP (adenosine triphosphate) from glucose and other energy-rich nutrients and this is used to drive other chemical reactions in the cell. During the first stage of cell respiration, glycolysis, which takes place in the cytoplasm, glucose is broken down into a simple molecule called pyruvate. This moves into the mitochondrion (*see* below/opposite) and is further broken down to release its energy which is transferred to the energy carrier ATP.

• **Ribosomes** are small granular organelles produced in the nucleolus. They are the site of protein synthesis, a key cellular activity described in more detail on pp. 8–9.

• **Endoplasmic reticulum** (ER) is a system of flattened, interconnected and folded membranes that acts as the cell's 'factory' by manufacturing, storing and transporting a range of substances. Rough ER is covered with ribosomes; proteins made by ribosomes are either stored here temporarily or are processed for export. Smooth ER lacks ribosomes and is involved in lipid synthesis.

• **Golgi complex** is a set of flattened, membrane sacs that resembles a stack of dinner plates. It processes proteins from rough ER and packages them in secretory vesicles that pinch off, migrate to the cell membrane and discharge their contents to the outside. Other vesicles remain in the cell as lysosomes.

• **Lysosomes** are small membrane-bound sacs that are filled with digestive enzymes. Their role is to digest worn-out organelles and foreign substances so their components can be recycled and reused.

• **Centrioles** are small, column-like organelles that occur in pairs at right angles to each other and which play a part in cell division.

• **Nucleus** is the cell's control centre and is separated from the cytoplasm by a double membrane, the nuclear envelope, which has pores. Its role in cell activities is described more fully on pp. 8–9.

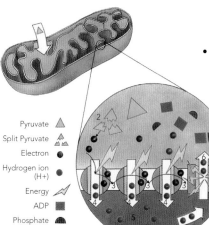

Pyruvate △
Split Pyruvate ⚠
Electron ●
Hydrogen ion (H+) ●
Energy ⚡
ADP ▰
Phosphate ▰
ATP ▰▶

▲ *The proton powerhouse*
Cells are powered primarily by energy released from ATP (adenosine triphosphate) as it becomes ADP (adenosine diphosphate). ATP is made in the mitochondria (1) by recycling ADP. Pyruvate (2) *is split into carbon dioxide, hydrogen and high-energy electrons. The electrons pass along a line of proteins in the inner membrane (3) providing energy to pump out protons (4) into the intermembrane space (5). As more protons are* *pumped out, pressure builds up, forcing protons back across the membrane. But the protons can only flow back into the matrix via the ATP generator (6) – the enzyme ATP synthetase – and produce ATP (7).*

HOW CELLS WORK

Cell chemistry

Inside a cell, a complex sequence of thousands of chemical reactions – collectively known as **metabolism** – takes place every second. Metabolism itself consists of two linked processes: anabolism and catabolism. **Anabolism** consists of those processes, such as protein synthesis, that manufacture substances needed by the cell to build or run itself. **Catabolism** consists of those processes, such as the breakdown of glucose during aerobic respiration, that release energy to power anabolism. Raw materials for both anabolism and catabolism are provided by nutrients absorbed from the small intestine following digestion.

Enzymes

These protein catalysts accelerate the rate of chemical reactions by thousands or millions of times – thereby making life possible – without being changed or consumed themselves. Each enzyme has a specific three-dimensional shape, and each is specific to a particular chemical reaction. Reactions are catalysed in part of the enzyme called the 'active site'.

Chromosomes and DNA

Chromosomes are long, thread-like structures located in the nucleus of every body cell. Most body cells are diploid, i.e. they contain two sets of chromosomes, with 23 chromosomes in each set (46 in all); 23 of the chromosomes are inherited from the person's mother (maternal) and 23 from their father (paternal). Chromosomes of the same size – one maternal and one paternal – form matching pairs, called homologous pairs. Sex cells – sperm and ova – are haploid: they each contain just one set of chromosomes. When they fuse during fertilization, the diploid chromosome number is restored.

Chromosomes are formed from deoxyribonucleic acid (DNA), a macromolecule unique in its ability to replicate

◀ **DNA** molecules form a double helix, with two spiral backbones (*1, 2*). These are made up of sugar and phosphate units. Linking the backbones are the bases: adenine (*3*), thymine (*4*), guanine (*5*) and cytosine (*6*). Each backbone contributes one base to each rung, which are paired; adenine with thymine and cytosine with guanine.

◀ This karyotype shows a full complement of 46 chromosomes from a female body cell. Normally chromosomes are long, thin and tangled. But just before cell division (see opposite) they become much shorter and thicker. It is at this stage that these chromosomes were photographed. The photograph was then cut up, and the chromosomes arranged as homologous pairs (one maternal and one paternal) according to their length. The pairs were then ordered according to size as shown here and numbered 1–23 from top left to bottom right. The final pair (23) are the female sex chromosomes, designated XX. In a male the sex chromosomes are XY (not shown here), with the Y chromosome being significantly shorter than the X.

itself. DNA consists of two intertwined spiralling strands that form a double helix similar in shape to a twisted ladder. The sides of the 'ladder' are formed by a sugar-phosphate backbone and its 'rungs' by pairs of linked bases of which there are four types: adenine (A), cytosine (C), guanine (G) and thymine (T). Within DNA, A only binds with T and C only binds with G. The DNA molecules inside one set of chromosomes (a genome) have about 25,000 sections, called genes. Each gene controls the production of a protein within the cell. Each protein has a specified use such as constructing cell components or making enzymes. By controlling protein synthesis, therefore, DNA controls all cell activities and all body features. Within genes, it is the precise but varying sequence of the bases A, C, G and T that provide the coded instructions used to make proteins. When cells divide (see below) during growth or repair, DNA duplicates itself exactly, so that each new cell has a precise copy of its parent cell's chromosomes, DNA and genes.

Protein synthesis

Proteins are made up of building blocks called amino acids, of which there are 20 different kinds. The functioning of a protein depends on its shape and this, in turn, depends on the precise order of amino acids in its molecule. During protein synthesis, the cell uses a genetic code to turn the instructions written in bases in the DNA of a gene to a sequence of amino acids in a protein. Each instruction is written in 'words', called codons, made of three 'letters', or bases, such as AAG. The first step, called transcription, is to copy the codons in a gene into a shorter, single-stranded molecule called messenger ribonucleic acid (often abbreviated as mRNA). This passes out of the nucleus and into the cytoplasm where the genetic message is translated (see below).

▶ *Translation Once in the cytoplasm, messenger ribonucleic acid (mRNA) attaches itself to a codon-reading machine called a ribosome. As the ribosome progresses along the mRNA, clover-leaf shaped molecules called transfer RNA or tRNA – of which there are many types – deliver their specific amino acid. Which amino acid they carry depends on the sequence of three bases – the anticodon – that projects from their base. The tRNA lines up with the complementary sequence of bases in the codon on mRNA. The amino acids link up through peptide bonds, and the DNA instructions have been successfully translated into an amino acid sequence.*

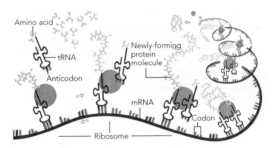

Amino acid

tRNA

Anticodon

Newly-forming protein molecule

mRNA

Ribosome

Codon

Chromosomes shorten and replicate

Chromosomes line up

Chromatids separate

Cell division completed

◀ *Mitosis This is the process, used in growth and repair, by which a cell nucleus divides to produce two identical cells. Each chromosome copies itself to form an X-shaped structure composed of two linked identical chromatids. Chromosomes line up in the centre of the cell and then the chromatids are pulled apart to each end of the cell, each forming a new chromosome. After mitosis, the cytoplasm divides to form two new cells.*

TISSUE, ORGANS, SYSTEMS

The human body is organized according to a hierarchy of levels of increasing structural complexity from the simplest (molecules) through cells (see pp. 6–7), tissues, organs and systems to the most complex, the body itself.

Tissues

Tissues are aggregations of cells of the same, or similar type, that are grouped together to perform a specific function, and collectively make up the fabric of the body. The study of tissues is known as histology. There are four main categories of tissues: epithelial, connective, muscle and nervous.

Epithelial tissue

Also called epithelium (pl. epithelia), epithelial tissues typically form linings inside the body, such as those of the mouth, fallopian tubes and blood vessels, as well as forming the skin's epidermis. Epithelial tissue consists of a continuous sheet of tightly packed cells, that may be one cell thick or have many cell layers and forms a leakproof barrier that prevents the admission of disease-causing microorganisms. It rests on, and is supported by, connective tissue (see below); between them is a basement membrane that reinforces the epithelial sheet by helping it resist tearing and stretching forces. They

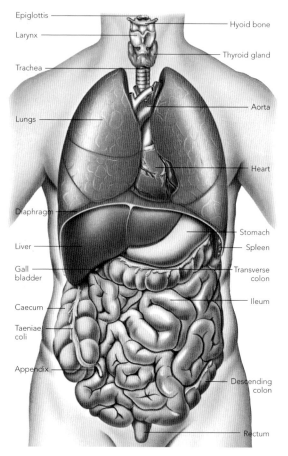

Epiglottis
Larynx
Trachea
Lungs
Diaphragm
Liver
Gall bladder
Caecum
Taeniae coli
Appendix

Hyoid bone
Thyroid gland
Aorta
Heart
Stomach
Spleen
Transverse colon
Ileum
Descending colon
Rectum

◄ *Cell, tissue, organ, system and body* This diagram illustrates the hierarchical organization of the body using the digestive system as an example. Four types of **cells** form the epithelial **tissue** that lines the stomach and secretes digestive juices. Epithelial tissue is just one of the tissues that makes up the J-shaped **organ** of the stomach, which is responsible for storing and partially digesting food. The stomach also contains smooth muscle that churns up food, nerve fibres that regulate the rate of muscle contraction and connective tissue that binds the other layers' tissues together. Stomach, small intestine and other linked organs form the digestive **system**, responsible for ingesting, digesting and absorbing food.

are classified in two ways. First, whether they consist of one layer (simple) or many layers (stratified) and second, by the shape of their cells – either squamous (flattened), cuboidal (box-like) or columnar (column-shaped).

Connective tissue

Connective tissues form the human body's framework by binding, supporting, strengthening and insulating other tissues. Uniquely, connective tissues consist principally of extracellular material (or matrix) secreted by widely scattered cells. This material has two components: ground substance and protein fibres. Ground substance fills the space between cells. It can be solid, fibrous, jelly-like, semi-fluid or fluid and contains fibres. Fibres include two main types: collagen fibres are tough and strong while elastin fibres stretch and recoil like rubber bands.

There are four main types of connective tissue. **Connective tissue proper** supports and binds other tissues: as adipose tissue, it stores fat for insulation and protection and it plays a role in tendons, ligaments and the skin's dermis. **Cartilage** is a tough but flexible structural tissue that has three forms: hyaline cartilage covers the ends of bones, elastic cartilage is found in the external ear and epiglottis and fibrous cartilage forms the intervertebral discs. **Bone**, with its hard matrix, supports the body and protects its internal organs. **Blood**, with its liquid matrix, is the transport medium of the cardiovascular system.

Connective and epithelial tissues combine to form the membranes that line body cavities and hollow organs. Cutaneous membrane forms the skin. Moist mucous membrane (mucosa) lines body cavities, such as the digestive system, that open to the outside. Serous membranes (serosa) cover and lubricate the walls of closed body cavities, such as the thoracic cavity, and the organs inside them and allow them to slide painlessly over each other.

Muscle tissue

Muscle tissue consists of well-vascularized cells, called fibres, that can contract, thereby causing movement. There are

three types of muscle tissue (see pp. 28–29): **skeletal muscle** moves and maintains the posture of the body, **smooth muscle** in the walls of hollow organs moves materials through the body and **cardiac muscle**, found only in the heart, pumps blood along the blood vessels.

Nervous tissue

Found only in the nervous system (see pp. 34–35), nervous tissue controls and regulates body functions. It consists of two types of cells: **neurons** generate and conduct nerve impulses at high speed and **glial cells** (or glia or neuroglia) support, protect and insulate neurons.

Organs and systems

An organ – such as the eye, heart or skin – is a structure that carries out a particular function or functions and is made up of two or more types of tissues. Linked organs – such as the brain, spinal cord, nerves and sense organs – form one of the 12 systems in the body, in this case the nervous system.

Systems

The body's 12 systems interact to form a complete, functioning human being. The integumentary system forms the body's external covering. The skeletal system supports the body, protects its organs and provides anchorage for skeletal muscles. The muscular system moves the body and maintains posture. The nervous system controls and regulates the body. The endocrine system secretes hormones that regulate processes such as growth and reproduction. The cardiovascular system transports nutrients, oxygen and other materials to body cells. The lymphatic system drains excess fluid from the tissues. The immune system defends the body against infection by utilizing white blood cells and chemicals in the blood, lymphatic system and tissues. The respiratory system takes oxygen into the body and removes carbon dioxide. The digestive system supplies the body with nutrients. The urinary system eliminates metabolic waste and regulates water balance. The reproductive systems (male and female) produce offspring.

Skin

Skin is the largest body organ. It weighs up to 5 kg (11 lb) and covers an area of about 2 sq m (21.5 sq ft), forming an interface between the body's interior and its surroundings. As a physical barrier, skin stops water from leaking out of or into the tissues, prevents the entry of bacteria and other disease-causing microorganisms, filters out the harmful and potentially carcinogenic ultraviolet (UV) radiation in sunlight and repairs itself if cut or torn. Skin also helps to maintain the body's temperature at a constant 37°C (98.6°F) and contains a range of sensory receptors (*see* pp. 46–47).

Skin structure

Skin has two layers: the epidermis and dermis. The **epidermis** is the thin, upper part of the skin. Its main role is protective. Its uppermost layer consists of dead, flattened cells, packed with keratin (a tough, waterproof protein), that are constantly worn away by everyday wear and tear, releasing scaly skin flakes: they are replaced by living cells in deeper layers that divide continuously. Other epidermal cells, called melanocytes, produce the brown pigment melanin, which gives skin its colour and forms a protective screen which absorbs harmful UV rays. People with darker skin produce more melanin; prolonged exposure to sunlight increases melanin production and temporarily darkens the skin.

The **dermis** is the lower, thicker part of the skin. A network of collagen and elastin fibres gives this connective tissue, respectively, strength and elasticity. The dermis contains blood vessels that play a part in temperature regulation (*see* opposite), sensory nerve endings and receptors that detect external stimuli, deep pits called hair follicles from which hairs grow and sebaceous glands that release an oily, bactericidal liquid called sebum that helps keep the skin and hairs soft, flexible and waterproof. Sweat glands release watery sweat onto the surface of the skin in warm conditions, from where it evaporates to

Section through the skin

Flattened, keratinized cells

Dividing epidermal cells and melanocytes

Sensory nerve ending

Nerve fibres

Blood vessel

Adipose (fat) cells

Sweat pore

Hair shaft

Epidermis

Dermis

Sebaceous gland

Hair follicle

Sweat gland

Hair erector muscle

cool the body. Adipose (fat) cells beneath the dermis help to insulate the body.

Hair

Except for the palms, soles, lips, nipples and parts of the external genitals, millions of hairs are distributed over the surface of the skin, with more than 100,000 on the scalp alone. Human hair has no insulatory role except on the scalp, where it also protects the skin from sunlight. Hair acts as a sensor and keeps dust out of the eyes and nose. Hairs are tubes of dead cells filled with keratin that grow upwards and above the surface of the skin from living, dividing cells in the base of hair follicles. Scalp hair grows at about 2 mm (0.08 in) a week for three to five years and is then pushed out by a newly growing hair. In men over 30, the male sex hormone testosterone can disrupt this cycle and cause male pattern baldness. Hair colour is dependent on melanin content; hair becomes white with age because of a lack of pigmentation. There are two types of body hair. Fine vellus hairs cover the bodies of children and women. Coarser terminal hairs are found in the scalp and eyebrows of all humans, in the armpits and pubic regions of adults and in the body and facial hair of adult males.

Nails

Nails are scaly extensions of the epidermis that cover and protect the upper, distal ends of the fingers and toes and aid gripping. A nail is made of dead cells packed with keratin and grows from living cells at its base at about 5 mm (0.2 in) per month (slower in toenails). Each nail consists of a free edge that projects from the tip of the finger or toe, a body covering the epidermis and coloured pink by the underlying dermis and a root embedded in the skin.

Proximal skin
fold or cuticle
Lunula
Body of nail

Nail bed

Free edge
of nail

Nail root

Nail matrix

Distal phalanx of finger

▲ *Section through nail*
The nail bed underlies the nail and consists of the deeper, living layer of the epidermis. At the proximal end of the nail bed is the thicker nail matrix. Nail growth happens as living cells in the nail matrix divide, push forwards and become keratinized to form the nail body, which slides over the nail bed. Much of the nail body appears pink, but a white crescent or lunula covers the nail matrix. Skin folds, called nail folds, overlap the proximal and lateral edges of the nails.

Hypothalamus

▲ *Temperature control*
The temperature centre in the hypothalamus controls heat loss and heat production by the body through the skin (below). Overheating (A) produces an increased blood flow from the blood vessels (1), which radiates heat and causes sweating through

the sweat glands (2), thereby losing heat. A fall in temperature (B) constricts the surface blood vessels, stops sweating and makes the erector muscles (3) contract, causing the hairs (4) to stand on end, thereby producing goose pimples. Additional heat can be produced by shivering.

THE SKELETON

The skeleton provides a strong, internal framework that supports the body, makes up about 20% of its weight, and consists of 206 bones. These bones meet at joints, the majority of which are freely moveable, making the skeleton flexible and mobile. The skeleton also contains cartilage and ligaments. **Cartilage** is a tough, flexible connective tissue that forms the frameworks of the ear and nose, links the ribs to the sternum and covers the ends of bones inside joints. **Ligaments** are strong strips of fibrous connective tissue that hold bones together at joints, thereby stabilizing the skeleton during movement. The bones of the skeleton are divided into two broad groups: the axial and appendicular skeletons.

Metacarpals
Carpals
Phalanges
Skull
Clavicle
Scapula
Costal cartilage
Sternum
Humerus
Rib
Vertebral column
(Backbone or spine)
Radius
Hip (pelvic
or coxal) bone
Ulna
Femur
Patella
Fibula
Tibia
Tarsals
Metatarsals
Phalanges

▶ *Axial skeleton This consists of 80 bones that form the body's long axis and are grouped into three regions: skull, vertebral column and ribcage. The skull is made up of 22 bones plus six ossicles, or ear bones, and, in the neck, the hyoid bone. The vertebral column consists of 26 irregular bones. The ribcage consists of 12 pairs of curved ribs linked to the sternum by flexible strips of costal cartilage. The axial skeleton serves to support the head, neck and trunk and protects the brain, spinal cord, lungs and heart.*

Other skeletal functions

In addition to supporting the body, the skeleton has other important functions. It surrounds and protects soft internal organs, such as the brain, heart and lungs, from external knocks and blows. It provides anchorage points for the tendons that link bones to skeletal muscles, which pull on bones across joints and move the body. Bones store the mineral calcium, which is needed for normal nerve and muscle function, releasing it into, or removing it from, the bloodstream according to the body's demands. Red bone marrow inside certain bones manufactures red and white blood cells. Yellow bone marrow inside long bones, such as the femur, stores fat.

Skull

Atlas
Axis

Cervical vertebrae

Clavicle
Pectoral girdle
Scapula

Humerus

Pelvic girdle

Radius

Ulna

Fibula

Tibia

Phalanges
Metacarpals
Carpals

Thoracic vertebrae

Lumbar vertebrae

Sacrum

Coccyx

Calcaneus (heel bone)

◄ *Appendicular skeleton*
The 126 bones of the appendicular skeleton make up the upper and lower extremities (limbs) and the girdles that attach them to the axial skeleton. Both upper and lower limbs consist of three sections. The upper limb consists of 27 hand bones, the radius and ulna (forearm bones) and the humerus (arm bone). The humerus articulates with a weak but very mobile pectoral girdle, consisting of the scapula and clavicle. The lower limb consists of 26 foot bones, the tibia and fibula (leg bones), the femur (thigh bone) and patella (kneecap). The femur articulates with a strong, almost rigid pelvic girdle made up of two hip bones.

BONE

Far from being dry and dusty, living bones are organs that are moist, have a rich supply of blood and lymph vessels and nerves and are constantly being reshaped. Bones are made of a hard connective tissue that consists of a matrix containing widely scattered bone cells called osteocytes. The matrix has two components. About 65% consists of mineral salts, especially calcium phosphate, which gives the bone hardness. Wrapped around these crystals is the fibrous protein collagen, which makes up about 35% of the matrix and gives some flexibility to bone. Together these elements make bone as strong as steel, but much lighter, and give it a degree of springiness that enables it to withstand the stresses gener-ated by supporting and moving the body without fracturing.

Inside bones

All bones are surrounded by periosteum, an outer protective 'skin' made of fibrous connective tissues through which pass the blood vessels that supply blood cells. Periosteum also contains cells that remodel bones in response to the stresses they experience: osteoclasts break cells down while osteoblasts build them up. Within the periosteum is a layer of com-pact, or cortical, tissue second only in hardness to tooth enamel. Compact bone consists of macroscopic cylinders of bone matrix called osteons that run in parallel, each acting as a weight-bearing

Spongy bone

Trabecula

Lamellae

Blood vessel

Osteon

Central (Haversian) canal

Canaliculi
Lacuna containing osteocyte

▲ **Compact and spongy bone** This section though a bone shows the outer compact bone and the inner spongy bone. The cylindrical osteons that make up compact bone consist of concentric tubes (lamellae) of matrix surrounding a central (Haversian) canal that carries blood vessels.

These supply widely spaced bone cells, called osteocytes, that are 'trapped' within spaces, called lacunae, found between the lamellae. Osteocytes communicate with each other through tiny 'tentacles' that pass along hair-like canals called canaliculi. Spongy bone consists of struts, called

trabeculae, made of irregularly arranged lamellae and osteocytes and spaces. Trabeculae are arranged along lines of stress, an arrangement that gives spongy bone considerable strength. The spaces make spongy bone much lighter than the compact bone that surrounds it.

pillar and collectively conferring great strength. Within compact bone is honeycomb-like spongy, or cancellous, bone. Despite its structure, spongy bone retains considerable strength, but its lightness reduces the overall weight of the skeleton. The spaces within spongy bone – and the central medullary cavity in long bones such as the femur – are filled with soft bone marrow. At birth, all bone marrow is red, the type that produces blood cells. By adulthood, red bone marrow in the long bones has been replaced by yellow marrow which provides a fat store.

Bone growth

Inside the uterus, the skeleton of the early fetus is made of hyaline cartilage. Gradually osteoblasts replace this cartilage framework with bone matrix. This process, known as ossification, continues from birth to adolescence. Osteoblasts develop growing bones from the outside and then become embedded within the matrix and change roles to become mature bone cells or osteocytes. In adulthood, although growth ceases, bones are constantly renewed, or remodelled, to strengthen those parts that are subjected to greatest stresses. Remodelling is achieved by the balanced activities of osteoclasts, which erode bone tissue, and osteoblasts, which rebuild it. Both osteoclasts and osteoblasts play a role in regulating levels of calcium in the blood.

Bone repair

Despite their strength, bones may break, or fracture, either as a result of extreme pressure caused by a fall or other accident or because of diseases such as osteoporosis. In a simple (closed) fracture, the broken ends of bones remain under the skin. In a compound (open) fracture, broken ends project out though the skin. As living tissue, bones have their own built-in repair system. Where possible, fractured bones need to be immobilized by a cast or, in more severe cases, by pinning, to ensure bones are correctly aligned as they heal.

Bone repair A fractured bone goes through several stages of repair before it is fully healed. Around six hours after the injury, a large haematoma (or blood clot) forms at the fracture site. This seals off any ruptured blood vessels and the site becomes inflamed. The periosteum regrows around the fracture site. Within days, capillaries grow into the haematoma, phagocytes move in to mop up debris, and the haematoma becomes replaced by a fibrous cartilage callus in which osteoblasts start to lay down new bone and hold two broken ends together. About four weeks after fracture, a bony callus of spongy bone forms. In the next few months, the bone is remodelled by osteoclasts to remove excess material on the bone's shaft and an outer layer of compact bone is laid down to complete the repair.

THE SKULL

The human skull shapes the head and face, protects the fragile brain and houses and protects the special sense organs for taste, smell, hearing, vision and balance. It is constructed from 22 bones, 21 of which are locked together by immovable joints, known as **sutures**, to form a structure of great strength. Blood vessels and cranial nerves enter and leave the skull through holes called **foramina** (sing. foramen) and canals. Skull bones divide into two groups: cranial bones and facial bones.

Cranial bones

The eight bones of the **cranium** support, surround and protect the brain within the cranial cavity. They form the roof, sides and back of the cranium, as well as the cranial floor on which the brain rests. The frontal bone forms the forehead, the anterior part of the cranial floor and the roof of the orbits (eye sockets). Two parietal bones form the roof and sides of the cranium. Two temporal bones form the inferior lateral parts of the cranium and part of the cranial floor. An opening in the temporal bone, the **external auditory meatus**, directs sounds into the inner part of the ear that is encased within, and which contains three small, linked bones called ossicles. The occipital bone forms the posterior part of the cranium and much of the cranial floor. The **occipital bone** has a large opening, the **foramen magnum**, through which the brain connects to the spinal cord. The **occipital condyles** articulate with the atlas (first cervical vertebra), enabling nodding movements of the head. The **ethmoid bone** forms part of the cranial floor, the medial walls of the orbits and the upper part of the nasal septum, which divides

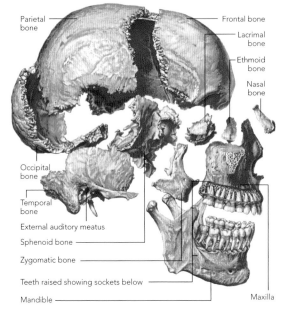

▶ *Skull bones This exploded view of the skull shows many of the component bones that make up its structure. The exposed edges of most bones, apart from the mandible, can be seen to have jagged or serrated edges. These edges fit together like pieces of a jigsaw to form immovable joints called sutures that are found only in the skull and which give it enormous strength and rigidity. The inner surface of the cranial bones is attached to the meninges (membranes) which surround, protect and stabilize the brain. Depressions in the inner* cranial surface accommodate blood vessels that supply the meninges. The outer surfaces of both cranial *and facial bones provide areas of attachment for muscles that move the head and produce facial expressions.*

Parietal bone
Frontal bone
Lacrimal bone
Ethmoid bone
Nasal bone
Occipital bone
Temporal bone
External auditory meatus
Sphenoid bone
Zygomatic bone
Teeth raised showing sockets below
Mandible
Maxilla

the nasal cavity vertically into left and right sides. The **sphenoid bone**, which is shaped like a bat's wings, acts as a keystone by articulating with, and holding together, all the other cranial bones.

Facial bones

The 14 facial bones form the framework of the face; provide cavities for the sense organs of smell, taste and vison; anchor the teeth; form openings for the passage of food, water and air and provide attachment points for the muscles that produce facial expressions. Two **maxillae** form the upper jaw, contain sockets for the 16 upper teeth and link all other facial bones apart from the mandible (lower jaw). Two **zygomatic bones**, or cheekbones, form the prominences of the cheeks and part of the lateral margins of the orbits. Two **lacrimal bones** form part of the medial wall of each orbit. Two **nasal bones** form the bridge of the nose. Two **palatine bones** form the posterior side walls of the nasal cavity and the posterior part of the

hard palate. Two inferior **nasal conchae** form part of the lateral wall of the nasal cavity. The **vomer** forms part of the nasal septum. The **mandible**, the only skull bone that is able to move, articulates with the temporal bone allowing the mouth to open and close and provides anchorage for the 16 lower teeth.

Sinuses

Sinuses are air-filled spaces found in the frontal, sphenoid, ethmoid and paired maxillae, clustered around the nasal cavity. These spaces reduce the overall weight of the skull.

Skull development

In the fetus, skull bones are formed by intramembranous ossification. A fibrous membrane ossifies to form skull bones linked by areas of as yet unossified membrane called **fontanelles**. At birth, these flexible areas allow the head to be slightly compressed and permit brain growth during early infancy.

Nasal bone
Orbit
Nasal cavity
Vomer
Inferior nasal concha
Mandible

Frontal bone
Parietal bone
Temporal bone
Sphenoid bone
Zygomatic bone
Maxilla

▲ **Front view of skull** Each orbit is a bony cavity formed from parts of seven interlocking bones: frontal, zygomatic, sphenoid, maxilla, ethmoid, lacrimal and palatine. The orbit encases and protects the eyeball, and provides attachment points

for the muscles that move the eye. The nasal cavity is formed from parts of the ethmoid, palatine, maxillae, vomer, inferior nasal conchae and by cartilage. It warms and moistens inhaled air and houses olfactory (smell) receptors.

Anterior fontanelle
Posterior fontanelle

▲ **Neonate skull** This skull of a newborn child shows two of the prominent fontanelles present at birth: the anterior fontanelle between the parietal and frontal bones and the posterior fontanelle between the parietal and occipital bones. Fontanelles are replaced by bone between one and two years after birth.

BACKBONE AND RIBS

Together with the sternum and ribs, the backbone (also known as the vertebral column, spinal column or spine) forms the skeleton of the trunk. The backbone consists of a chain of irregular bones called **vertebrae** that meet at slightly movable joints. Each joint permits only limited movement, but collectively the joints give the backbone considerable flexibility enabling it to rotate and to bend anteriorly, posteriorly and laterally. The average backbone makes up about 40% of body height. It extends from the skull to its anchorage in the pelvic girdle, where it transmits the weight of the head and trunk to the lower limbs. It also supports the skull, encloses and protects the delicate spinal cord and provides attachment points for the ribs and for the muscles and ligaments that support the trunk of the body.

Intervertebral discs
Intervertebral discs are found between adjacent vertebrae from the second cervical vertebra (axis) to the sacrum. Each disc has an inner soft, pulp nucleus covered by an outer covering of fibrous cartilage. Each disc forms a strong, slightly movable joint. Collectively, discs cushion vertebrae against vertical shocks and allow various movements of the backbone.

Vertebral curves
Seen in side view (left) a normal backbone has four curves that give it an S shape. The cervical and lumbar curves are convex anteriorly while the thoracic and sacral curves are concave anteriorly. The S shape allows the backbone to function as a spring rather than a flexible rod, thereby absorbing shock during walking and running, enhancing the strength and flexibility of the backbone and facilitating balance when upright by placing the trunk directly over the feet.

Bony thorax
The cone-shaped bony thorax surrounds the thoracic cavity, and is formed by 12

Atlas
Axis
Cervical vertebrae
1
1 Cervical curve
2 Thoracic curve
3 Lumbar curve
4 Sacral curve
2
Thoracic vertebrae
Intervertebral disc
Lumbar vertebrae
3
Sacrum
4
Coccyx

◀ *Regions of the backbone An adult backbone consists of 26 vertebrae of which two, the sacrum and coccyx, are composites consisting of vertebrae that fused during childhood. The backbone has five sections. Seven small cervical vertebrae form the neck, the most flexible part of the backbone. The uppermost cervical vertebra, the atlas, articulates with the occipital condyle of the skull to enable nodding 'Yes' movements of the head;* *articulation of the atlas with the axis, the second cervical vertebra, produces shaking 'No' movement of the head. Each of the 12 thoracic vertebrae articulates with a pair of ribs. Five large lumbar vertebrae form the hollow small of the back and bear most of the weight of the head and trunk. The triangular sacrum, made of five fused bones, forms a strong anchorage for the pelvic girdle, with which it forms the pelvis. The coccyx, or tailbone, consists of four fused vertebrae.*

Structure of vertebrae
The anterior pillar-like centrum, or body, bears the weight of the trunk and head. Attached to the centrum posteriorly is the ring-shaped vertebral, or neural, arch: between the two is the vertebral foramen. Successive vertebral foramina of adjacent vertebrae form the vertebral canal which encases and protects the spinal cord. Projecting posteriorly from the vertebral arch is a spinous process, and laterally two transverse processes. These provide attachment points for the muscles and ligaments that stabilize the backbone. Paired superior and inferior articular processes bear smooth joint surfaces, called facets, that form movable joints with adjacent vertebrae, in addition to the joints formed by intervertebral discs.

thoracic vertebrae posteriorly, 12 pairs of ribs laterally and the sternum and costal cartilages anteriorly. Its cage-like structure protects the thoracic and upper abdominal organs, supports the pectoral girdles and upper limbs and plays a part in breathing.

Ribs

The ribs are curved, flat bones with a slightly twisted shaft. The 12 pairs of ribs form a ribcage that protects the heart, lungs, major blood vessels, stomach and liver. At its posterior end, the head of each rib articulates with the facets on the centra of adjacent vertebrae and with a facet on a transverse process. These vertebrocostal joints are plane joints that allow gliding movements. At their anterior ends, the upper ten pairs of ribs attach directly or indirectly to the sternum by flexible costal cartilages. Ribs 11 and 12 have no anterior attachments: their costal cartilages are embedded in the abdominal wall. Together, vertebrocostal joints and costal cartilages give the ribcage sufficient flexibility to make movements up and down during breathing. Such movements are achieved by intercostal muscles (see p. 78)

▶ *Ribcage The 12 pairs of ribs in the ribcage increase in size up to the seventh pair, and then they decrease. The seven superior pairs of ribs, known as the true or vertebrosternal ribs, attach directly to the sternum through their own costal cartilages. The remaining five pairs of ribs are called false ribs. The costal cartilages of the eighth to tenth pairs, the vertebrochondral ribs, attach to each other and to the costal cartilage of the*

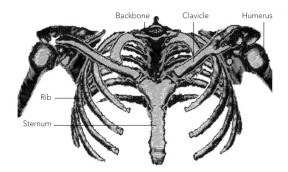

seventh pair of ribs. These costal cartilages form the inferior, or costal, margin of the ribcage. The eleventh and twelfth ribs, the floating or vertebral ribs, have no anterior attachment to the sternum.

21

THE SHOULDER AND ARM

Unlike their close relatives in the animal kingdom, humans have an upright stance and walk on their hind limbs or lower limbs. This leaves their forelimbs – the upper limbs – free to pick up and manipulate objects. The bones of the shoulder and arm are, accordingly, thinner and more mobile than the stronger weight-bearing bones of the lower limbs.

Pectoral girdle

The pectoral, or shoulder, girdle is formed on each side of the body by two bones: the **clavicle**, or collarbone, and the **scapula**, or shoulder blade. Together, these two bones and their associated muscles form the shoulder. The pectoral girdle attaches the upper limb to the trunk and provides anchorage points for the muscles that move the upper limb. Unlike the pelvic (hip) girdle, the pectoral girdle is light and highly mobile and it is not attached to the backbone. The long, curved clavicle articulates with the sternum at its medial end and scapula at its lateral end. It acts as strut which holds the scapula and arm away from the upper part of the thorax. The triangular scapula lies on the dorsal surface of the ribcage. Its lateral margin, next to the armpit, forms a shallow, cup-like cavity, the glenoid cavity. The head of the humerus fits into the glenoid cavity to form a ball and socket joint, the shoulder joint. This joint is highly mobile, but not very stable, because the glenoid cavity is shallow and poorly reinforced and does not restrict the movement of the humerus.

Upper limb

The upper limb consists of 30 bones organized into three sections: the arm, forearm and hand. The **humerus**, the single bone of the arm and the largest

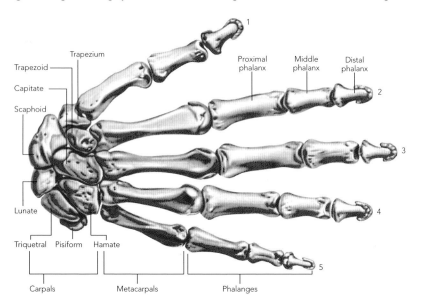

Trapezium
Trapezoid
Capitate
Scaphoid

Proximal phalanx
Middle phalanx
Distal phalanx

1
2
3
4
5

Lunate

Triquetral Pisiform Hamate

Carpals

Metacarpals

Phalanges

▲ **The hand** Hand bones fall into three groups. Arranged in two rows, eight short carpal bones form the wrist, which forms a flexible bridge between forearm and palm. Five metacarpal bones radiate from the wrist to form the palm of the hand. Their distal ends form the knuckles. Fourteen long bones called phalanges (sing. phalanx) form the digits, or fingers. Each finger has three phalanges – proximal, middle and distal – while the pollex, or thumb, has two.

and longest in the upper limb, articulates proximally with the scapula at the shoulder joint and distally in a hinge joint with the forearm bones, the **ulna** and **radius**, at the elbow. Running parallel in the forearm, the radius and ulna articulate distally with **carpals** in the wrist to form the wrist joint. At their proximal end they articulate with each other at a pivot joint, which allows the radius to cross over the ulna thereby enabling the hand to rotate through 180°. Each hand consists of 27 small bones that form the most flexible and versatile part of the skeleton which is strong enough to grip objects firmly and precise enough to write a letter, yet delicate enough to thread a needle.

▲ **The opposable thumb** A highly flexible saddle joint between the metacarpal of the thumb and the trapezium (a carpal) makes the thumb the most mobile of the digits. The thumb can swing across the palm and touch the tips of the other fingers in turn, an action called opposition. The opposable thumb enables the hand to grip, including the precise grip shown in this X-ray.

Humerus

Ulna

Radius

Carpals

Metacarpals

Phalanges

Clavicle

Scapula

Glenoid cavity

Humerus

▲ **Shoulder and arm** The arrangement of bones in the shoulder, arm and hand provides great flexibility and a wide range of movement. The arm can be extended forwards to grasp objects, then folded back against the body. It can also move out to the side, upwards and backwards and swing around.

▲ **Shoulder joint** Clearly visible here are the bones that form the shoulder joint. The ball-like upper end of the humerus fits into the shallow glenoid cavity of the scapula to form a highly mobile but unstable joint.

23

Pelvic girdle

The pelvic, or hip, girdle is the strong, rigid structure which attaches the legs to the trunk and transmits the weight of the upper body to the legs. It consists of two **coxal**, or hip, bones which meet anteriorly at the pubic symphysis and posteriorly are firmly connected to the **sacrum**.

Hip bones

Each hip bone is made up of three fused bones: the ilium, ischium and pubis. The **ilium** forms the largest part of the hip bone. Posteriorly, each ilium articulates with the sacrum at the sacroiliac joint through which the weight of the upper body is transmitted from the backbone to the pelvic girdle. The L-shaped **ischium**, which is inferior and posterior, bears a person's weight when they sit. The **pubis**, or pubic bone, is anterior and is linked to its partner by a fibrous cartilage disc to form a slightly moveable joint. Where the three bones meet on the lateral surface of each hip bone, they form a deep, cup-like socket called the **acetabulum** into which fits the ball-like head of the **femur** (thigh bone) at

Anterior view of the pelvis

Hip bones
This view of the pelvis – shown as if lying down – shows the two fused hip bones that make up the pelvic girdle. The hip bone has three component bones, the ilium, ischium and pubis. Separate during childhood, the three bones fuse during adolescence. Also seen clearly here is the acetabulum, or socket, that houses the head of the femur in the hip joint.

Male pelvis   Female pelvis

▲ **Male and female pelvis**
The male and female pelvis show clear differences. The male pelvis is made of heavier, thicker, bones and is narrow and deep. It has a narrow, long sacrum, a narrow pubic arch (the inverted V-shaped arch that is inferior to the pubic symphysis) and a pelvic *inlet (the central opening of the pelvis) that is narrow and heart shaped. The male pelvis is adapted to support the male's heavier build and stronger muscles. The female pelvis is broader and shallower than the male pelvis. It has a wide short sacrum, a broad pubic arch and a pelvic* *inlet that is wide and round. This structure reflects the female's role in childbearing. The broader pelvis supports the fetus during its development. The pelvic inlet is wide enough to allow the fetus's relatively large head to pass through it during childbirth.*

the hip joint. This ball-and-socket joint allows less freedom of movement than the one found in the shoulder between the humerus and pectoral girdle because of the strong ligaments that constrain it. However, although less mobile, the hip joint is much more stable than the shoulder joint.

Lower limb

The lower limb consists of 30 bones organized into three sections: the thigh, leg and

◄ Hip and femur
The femur and acetabulum fit together forming a ball-and-socket joint that allows for articulation.

Coxal (hip) bone
Acetabulum
Head of femur
Femur

▼ Hip and leg
Linked to the rest of the body through the pelvic girdle, the lower limbs support the entire weight of the body and withstand the considerable forces generated during walking, running, or jumping. These roles are reflected in the fact that the lower limb bones are much stronger and thicker than those that make up the upper limb.

Coxal (hip) bone
Hip joint
Femur
Knee joint
Tibia
Fibula

foot. The thigh bone, or **femur**, is the body's longest and strongest bone and bears its weight. At its proximal end, its rounded head forms the hip joint with the acetabulum of the pelvic girdle. Where its laterally angled neck joins the long shaft, there are projections called **trochanters** to which thigh and buttock muscles attach. At its distal end the femur widens into two condyles to form the knee joint with the proximal end of the tibia. The triangular **patella**, or kneecap, protects the knee joint anteriorly. The leg has two parallel bones, the tibia and fibula. The **tibia** transmits the body's weight from femur to foot. At its distal end it forms a hinge joint – the ankle joint – with the talus, one of the tarsal bones in the foot. The slender **fibula** articulates at both ends with the tibia and adds stability to the leg. The broad feet bear the body's weight, help to keep it balanced during movement and when stationary and act as levers that push the body forwards during movement.

Pelvis

Together, the pelvic girdle and sacrum form the pelvis. Reinforced by strong ligaments, the basin-shaped pelvis supports the abdominal organs and surrounds and protects the organs of the lower abdomen including the reproductive organs and the urinary bladder. It also provides anchorage for powerful muscles that move the legs and support the trunk.

Tarsals
Metatarsals
Phalanges

▲ Foot bones
The foot is made up of 26 bones in all. Seven tarsal bones form the ankle. Five metatarsals form the sole of the foot which, reinforced by ligaments and tendons, forms a spring-like arch that absorbs impact during walking and running. The 14 phalanges form the toes, and are less mobile than those in the fingers. The arrangement of the bones in the foot allow little free movement compared to the hand but enable the foot to act as a weight bearer and mover.

JOINTS

A joint, or articulation, is a part of the skeleton where two or more bones meet. Joints allow the skeleton to move. They also hold the skeleton together and give it stability because the bones in a joint are held together by strips of tough fibrous connective tissue called ligaments. In all joints, the ends of bones do not touch directly but are separated by layers of cartilage or fibrous tissue. Joints can be classified into three types – fixed, slightly moveable and moveable joints – according to the amount of movement they permit. The more moveable a joint is, the less strength it has.

Fixed joints
Fixed (immoveable) joints permit no movement. The most obvious example of this type of joint are the sutures that, like seams, connect the bones of the skull. In a suture, the serrated edges of skull bones lock together like pieces of a jigsaw, reinforced by fibrous tissue between them. This arrangement gives the skull great strength, vital for its role of protecting the brain.

Slightly moveable joints
This type of joint allows a small amount of movement, and provides strength with flexibility. Typically, the articular surface of the bone is covered with hyaline cartilage which is fused to a pad of compressible fibrous cartilage which separates the two bones and permits limited movement. In the backbone, for example, slightly moveable joints between adjacent vertebrae allow limited movement, but collectively all the movement of all vertebrae give the backbone considerable flexibility. A further example of this type of joint is the pubic symphysis in the anterior part of the pelvis.

Moveable joints
Moveable, or synovial, joints allow bones to move freely, make up most of the joints in the skeleton and enable the body to perform a wide range of movements including walking, chewing and writing. While there are different types of moveable joints, each with its own range of movement, all have the same basic structure which allows free movement yet also provides stability. Inside the joint, opposing bone surfaces are covered by glassy hyaline (articular) cartilage, a hard-wearing coat that reduces friction between bones when they move and helps to absorb shocks during movement, thereby pre-

Types of moveable human joints
These illustrations show the range of movements permitted by six main types of moveable joints in the body. In most the bones hinge on each other or rotate. In the plane joint the bones glide over each other.

Saddle joint
Two U-shaped surfaces allow movement in two directions and in a circle. Found at the base of the thumb.

Hinge joint
Allows movement in one plane, e.g. flexion and extension of knee or elbow.

Plane joint
Allows bones to make small sliding movements from side to side, e.g. tarsal bones in foot.

Condyloid joint
Allows movement in two directions and in a circle, e.g. knuckle joint.

Ball and socket joint Allows movement in many directions, e.g. shoulder and hip joints.

Pivot joint Allows rotation, but no other movement, e.g. between the atlas and axis.

venting bone ends from being crushed. Between the cartilage-covered bone ends there is a space called the synovial, or joint, cavity. This is enclosed by the articular, or joint, capsule. Its outer layer is a

▼ *Moveable joint* This section though the knee joint shows the main parts of a moveable joint. The fatty pad, found in knee and hip joints, has a cushioning effect.

— Femur

— Patellar ligament

— Hyaline cartilage

— Fatty pad

— Joint cavity

— Tibia

— Muscle

tough fibrous coat that strengthens the joint by holding the bones together. Its inner layer is the synovial membrane that secretes an oily, yellow liquid, called synovial fluid, into the synovial cavity. Synovial fluid reduces friction further by making the hyaline cartilage more slippery, thereby increasing ease of movement. Moveable joints are reinforced by ligaments external to the joint capsule: some, including the knee, have internal ligaments to provide additional reinforcement. The muscles that pass across a joint and link bones on either side of it also play a part in stabilizing it. Some moveable joints, such as the knee, have wedges of fibrous cartilage called articular discs, or **menisci** (sing. meniscus), separating articular surfaces. They improve the fit between bones ends, thereby both reducing wear and tear and stabilizing the joint.

Moveable joints are divided into six types – plane, hinge, pivot, condyloid, saddle and ball-and-socket joints – according to the shapes of the articular surfaces of component bones, and the range of movement they allow. The degree of movement of a particular joint is also affected by how tightly ligaments hold the bones together.

▶ *The knee joint* is the largest and most complex joint in the body. As it reaches full extension it rotates slightly and 'locks' into a rigid limb from hip to ankle, helped by the bony protuberances at the lower end of the femur and the two semilunar cartilages attached to the sides of the upper end of the tibia. The ligaments surrounding the joint are combined with the cruciate ligaments to prevent overextension. The tendon of the quadriceps femoris muscle surrounds the patella bone in front of the knee. This helps to protect the joint. Behind some tendons and ligaments there are bursae.

— Patella

Cruciate — ligament

Medial — ligament

— Lateral meniscus

— Lateral ligament

Medial — meniscus

Patellar — ligament

Tibia —

— Fibula

MUSCLES

Muscles produce movement of, and inside, the body. Muscle tissue is made up of cells called fibres that have the ability to contract, or shorten, in order to produce a pulling force. Muscles are extensible, so that they can be stretched, and elastic, allowing them to recoil and resume their normal resting length. Muscles are also electrically excitable, so that they can be stimulated to contract by a nerve impulse. Three types of muscle – skeletal, smooth and cardiac – are found in the body.

Skeletal muscle

As their name suggests, skeletal muscles are attached to the bones of the skeleton. There are more than 640 individually named muscles that together make up more than 40% of body weight and give the body its shape. They are arranged in layers that overlap each other. Those just below the skin are called superficial (see below) while those below the superficial muscle are called deep.

Typically each muscle attaches to two or more bones by tough cords of connective

Superficial skeletal muscles

Flexor retinaculum
Frontalis
Temporalis
Orbicularis oculi
Masseter
Orbicularis oris
Sternocleidomastoid
Serratus anterior
External oblique
Deltoid
Pectoralis major
Biceps brachii
Triceps brachii
Pronator teres
Sartorius
Quadriceps femoris
Flexor carpi radialis
Brachioradialis
Patella
Tibialis anterior

Extensor retinaculum
Occipitalis
Trapezius
Latissimus dorsi
Gluteus maximus
Semitendinosus
Biceps femoris
Semimembranosus
Gastrocnemius
Achilles' tendon

tissue known as **tendons**. When skeletal muscles contract across joints, they pull bones, producing a range of movements from running to chewing. Instructions for contraction come from the brain and spinal cord. Skeletal muscle is also known as **voluntary muscle** because a person can make a conscious decision to move their body, although under normal circumstances general body movements occur without conscious involvement. Skeletal muscles also maintain body posture by remaining in a state of partial contraction (tonus) that holds the body upright, stabilize and strengthen certain joints including the knee and shoulder and generate heat during contraction that is used to help maintain body temperature at 37°C (98.6°F).

Types of muscles

Cardiac muscle

Smooth muscle

Skeletal muscle

Smooth muscle

Smooth muscle occurs mainly in the walls of hollow organs where it controls, for example, the movement of food along the small intestine or the diameter of a blood vessel. It is also known as **involuntary muscle** because its contraction is triggered by nerve impulses from the autonomic nervous system (ANS) and its actions occur without conscious awareness or intervention. In many organs, it forms a double layer with sheets of smooth muscle fibres running at right angles to each other – longitudinal on the outside and circular on the inside. Innervation of the different layers by the opposing parts of the ANS (sympathetic and parasympathetic) causes opposite effects on the organ.

Cardiac muscle

Cardiac muscle is found solely in the wall of the heart. Its fibres do not require stimulation to contract: they do so automatically, regularly and without fatiguing, for a lifetime. Electrical impulses from part of the heart, called the pacemaker, travel across and though the heart wall and set the pace of contraction of other cardiac muscle fibres. The sympathetic and parasympathetic branches of the ANS respectively increase or decrease the rate set by the pacemaker in order to meet the human body's changing demands.

Section of muscle fibre

Muscle made of bundles of fibres

Branched muscle fibres

Spiral muscle

Circular muscle

Single muscle fibres

Longitudinal muscle

▲ *Skeletal muscles are made up of hundreds or thousands of cylindrical fibres, up to 30 cm (12 in) long, that have a striped (or striated) appearance under the microscope. They are bound together in bundles by connective tissue. They can contract rapidly and powerfully but fatigue (tire) easily.*

▲ *Cardiac muscle fibres, like skeletal muscle fibres, have a striped (or striated) appearance under the microscope, but are shorter and have branches which link up to form interconnected strands. They interweave to form a spiral band around the ventricles of the heart.*

▲ *Smooth muscle fibres are spindle-shaped – wide in the middle and tapering at each end – and are packed together in sheets. They lack the striations seen in other muscle fibres, hence the name 'smooth'. Smooth muscles contract slowly and rhythmically under the control of the autonomic nervous system.*

SKELETAL MUSCLE – MOVEMENT

Skeletal muscles move the body by pulling the bones that make up the skeleton across the moveable joints that connect them.

Muscle attachment

Each skeletal muscle is anchored to bones at two or more points by **tendons**. Many tendons are cord-like while others, called aponeuroses, are broader and sheet-like. Tendons are fashioned from connective tissue containing closely packed bundles of tough collagen fibres that run in parallel to the direction of pull and provide great tensile strength. The collagen fibres extend through a bone's periosteum (outer membrane) and are firmly embedded in the outer layer of compact bone. Typically, a muscle is attached to two bones: one, the **origin**, remains fixed during contraction; the other, the **insertion**, moves towards the origin bone.

Muscle interactions

Muscles pull but cannot push. When a muscle contracts to produce movement in one direction, there must be another muscle that causes movement in the opposite direction. Skeletal muscles are organized in groups or teams that produce a particular movement or movements. Within teams there are four functional groups of muscles: prime movers, antagonists, synergists and fixators. A **prime mover**, or agonist, provides the major force for movement, such as the biceps brachii flexing the arm at the elbow. An **antagonist**, such as the triceps brachii which extends the arm at the elbow, opposes the movement produced by the prime mover. **Synergists** assist prime movers by adding some extra force to the movement. **Fixators** are muscles that immobilize a bone or muscle origin, stabilizing that part of the body while other muscles are contracting.

Muscles, bones and levers

In terms of basic mechanics, a lever is a rigid bar that moves on a fixed point, called the fulcrum or pivot, when a force, or effort, is applied to it in order to move a weight or load, a principle used in many everyday tools. In biomechanical terms, muscles and bones interact to move the body using lever systems: bones are levers, a joint is a fulcrum and muscles provide the force to move the load produced by the weight of a body part. Levers fall into three classes according to the relative position of the force, fulcrum and weight.

First-class lever

The fulcrum lies between the force and the weight, as in a seesaw. Posterior neck muscles (force) pull the head (weight) up from the chest pivoted on the joint between occipital condyle and atlas (fulcrum).

Second-class lever

The weight lies between the force and the fulcrum, as in a wheelbarrow. When a person stands on tiptoe, the calf muscles (force) lift the body (weight), pivoting on the ball of the feet (fulcrum).

Third-class lever

The weight is applied to the lever between the force and the fulcrum, as in a pair of tweezers. During arm flexion, the biceps brachii (force) lifts the forearm (weight), pivoting on the elbow (fulcrum). This is the most common lever system in the body.

Range of movements

What type of movement, or movements, a muscle produces depend on its location, the type of joint or joints it crosses and the other muscles it works with. Specific terms are used to describe the movements produced by muscles and bones, as outlined below.

Flexion and extension

Flexion involves decreasing the angle between two bones, such as the bending of the arm at the elbow. Extension is the opposite action, increasing the angle between two bones, such as the straightening of the arm at the elbow.

Abduction and adduction

Abduction is the movement of a bone away from the body's midline, such as

Scapula

Triceps brachii contracted

Biceps brachii relaxed

Arm extended at the elbow

Biceps brachii contracted

Triceps brachii relaxed

Arm flexed at the elbow

Opposing muscles The biceps brachii and the triceps brachii in the upper limb provide a clear example of how muscles interact with bones to produce movement. Like all prime movers and antagonists, the biceps and triceps are located on either sides of the joint, in this case the hinge joint in the elbow. The biceps brachii has its origin in the scapula and insertion in the radius. The triceps has its origin in the scapula and humerus and insertion in the ulna. The biceps, prime mover of elbow flexion, contracts and pulls the forearm upwards towards the shoulder and its antagonist, the triceps, relaxes. When the triceps, the prime mover of elbow extension, contracts, it moves the forearm downwards, while its antagonist, the biceps, relaxes. The brachioradialis acts as a synergist to the biceps.

moving the arm laterally and upwards. Adduction is the opposite action, moving a bone towards the body's midline, such as moving the arm medially and downwards.

Elevation and depression

Elevation is an action that involves lifting upwards, i.e. the lifting of the lower jaw (mandible) in order to close the mouth. Depression is the opposite action; a downwards movement, such as opening the mouth.

Rotation and circumduction

Rotation involves a bone swivelling on its own axis, such as turning the head. Circumduction involves describing a circular movement with the upper or lower limb.

HOW MUSCLES CONTRACT

Skeletal muscles contract when they receive a nerve impulse from the brain or spinal cord. Contraction is caused by an interaction of protein filaments packed in parallel and in an orderly manner inside muscle fibres (cells). Contraction involves a transformation of chemical energy stored in nutrients, notably glucose, into kinetic (movement) energy, with a concomitant release of heat energy which contributes towards the maintenance of human body temperature at 37°C (98.6°F).

Skeletal muscle structure

Skeletal muscle consists of hundreds or thousands of long fibres, each between 0.001 mm and 0.1 mm (0.00004 and 0.004 in) and in diameter and up to 30 cm (12 in) in length, that run in parallel along the length of the muscle. Groups of fibres are grouped together in bundles, called **fascicles**, by an outer layer of connective tissue called **perimysium**. Fascicles, in turn, are bound together by a protective connective tissue sheath, called the **epimysium**, to form a complete muscle. A muscle fibre has a highly organized structure that reflects its unique contractile role. Each fibre is packed with thousands of rod-like **myofibrils** that run in parallel along the fibre. Myofibrils contain two types of protein filaments – thick **myosin** filaments and thin **actin** filaments – that are arranged in repeating units called **sarcomeres**. Within each sarcomere, filaments run in parallel and overlap. This arrangement gives myofibrils and fibres a striated, or striped, appearance when seen under the microscope.

Muscle contraction

Contraction occurs when the actin and myosin filaments slide over each other. This action requires energy provided in the form of adenosine triphosphate (ATP) released by aerobic respiration inside mitochondria. Inside each sarcomere, myosin filaments are arranged centrally; while actin filaments are attached to the vertical boundary at each end of the sarcomere, called the Z line. Extending from each myosin filament are 'heads' that, at rest, project towards but do not touch overlapping actin filaments. These heads are 'charged' with ATP. When a muscle

Epimysium
Perimysium
Muscle fibre
Myofibril
Sarcomere
Z line
Myofibril
Thick (myosin) filament
Thin (actin) filament

▶ **Inside a muscle** This schematic artwork reveals the hierarchical structure of a skeletal muscle by first sectioning the muscle and then projecting from its cut surface its component muscle fibres, from them the myofibrils that make up the fibres and finally the protein filaments that are packed inside the myofibrils.

fibre is stimulated to contract by a nerve impulse, the myosin head extends towards and touches the actin filament to form a cross bridge. Then, the head uses ATP energy to swivel towards the centre of the sarcomere, thereby pulling the acting filament inwards. It then breaks away, is recharged with ATP, and makes another cross bridge. This happens repeatedly making the myobril – and therefore the muscle fibre – shorter, until the nerve impulses cease, the cross bridges stop forming and the muscle fibre relaxes.

Neurons and muscles

Muscles are stimulated to contract by electrical nerve impulses that travel from the central nervous system along neurons (nerve cells) bundled together in nerves. Where a motor neuron approaches a muscle, it divides into several branches, called **axon terminals**, each of which serves a single muscle fibre. The motor neuron and muscle fibre meet at a neuromuscular junction, within which the two are separated by a tiny opening, called a **synaptic gap**. Arrival of nerve impulses causes release of a chemical neurotransmitter from the synaptic bulb at the end of the axon terminal. It passes across the

▼ *SEM of a neuromuscular junction. Axon terminals of the axon (nerve fibre) of a neuron (green) form synapses with muscle fibres (red).*

Motor neuron   Axon terminal   Muscle fibre

gap to the motor end plate, a folded region of the **sarcolemma** (cell membrane of the muscle fibre). Arrival of the neurotransmitter causes an electrical impulse to pass along the sarcolemma. This, in turn, triggers the formation of cross bridges by myosin and the contraction of the myofibril. Together, each motor neuron and the muscle fibres it supplies is called a motor unit. When a neuron fires it stimulates all the fibres in its motor unit to contract. The more neurons that fire, the more motor units are stimulated and the stronger the contraction of that particular muscle.

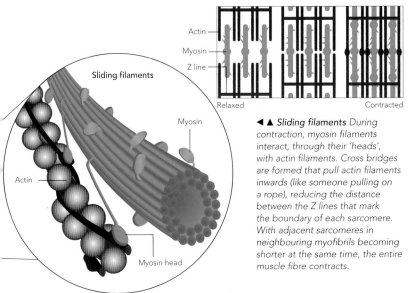

Actin
Myosin
Z line

Sliding filaments

Myosin

Actin

Myosin head

Relaxed   Contracted

◀ ▲ **Sliding filaments** *During contraction, myosin filaments interact, through their 'heads', with actin filaments. Cross bridges are formed that pull actin filaments inwards (like someone pulling on a rope), reducing the distance between the Z lines that mark the boundary of each sarcomere. With adjacent sarcomeres in neighbouring myofibrils becoming shorter at the same time, the entire muscle fibre contracts.*

NERVOUS SYSTEM

The nervous system is the human body's primary communication system which, together with the endocrine system (see pp. 56–57), controls and co-ordinates almost all body activities. Working day and night, it receives information from both outside and inside the body, gathered by sensors such as the eyes and proprioceptors; processes and, where appropriate, stores that information and sends out instructions to effectors, such as muscles and glands, to make the body react. The incredible speed and processing power of the nervous system means that it can cope with a wide range of tasks at the same time. It can, for example, enable a person to think, create, remember and feel while, unnoticed, it regulates a host of internal events such as heart rate or body temperature in order to help maintain **homeostasis** – the state of constancy, balance and stability that normally exists within a healthy body, regardless of external and internal changes.

Parts of the nervous system

The **central nervous system** (CNS) and **peripheral nervous system** (PNS) are outlined below (see diagram). The PNS has two parts. Its sensory division gathers information from sensors about changes inside and outside the body and transmits it to the CNS. Its motor division carries signals from the CNS to muscles and glands, and itself has two parts: the **somatic nervous system** instructs skeletal muscles to contract, enabling the body to respond consciously, and the **autonomic nervous system** or ANS (see pp. 44–45) automatically regulates internal processes, such as breathing and digestion, by transmitting instructions to the body's internal organs.

Nerve cells

The nervous system is made up of trillions of nerve cells, divided into two main groups: neurons and glia. **Neurons** are long, thin cells that generate and transmit

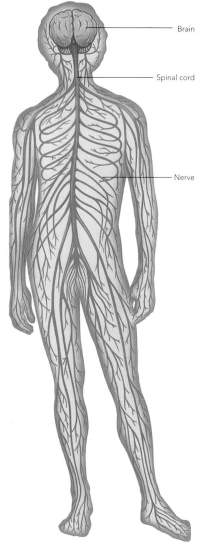

Brain

Spinal cord

Nerve

◀ *The nervous system This is divided into two main parts. The central nervous system (CNS) consists of the brain and spinal cord; these form the command centre of the nervous system and carry out the roles of processing and integration. The peripheral nervous system (PNS) consists of the cable-like nerves (bundles of sensory and motor neurons) that extend from the brain and spinal cord and relay messages between all parts of the body and the CNS.*

electrical signals called nerve impulses, and which together form a vast, high-speed communication system. There are three types of neurons. **Sensory neurons** conduct impulses generated when receptors – such as those in the skin, eyes or muscles – are stimulated to the CNS. **Motor neurons** carry nerve impulses from the CNS to muscles and glands. **Association neurons** or interneurons, which make up 90% of all neurons, are found inside the CNS: they link sensory and motor neurons and enable the CNS to sort and process information. **Glia** (or glial cells), also called neuroglia, support and nurture neurons.

Synapses

A synapse is a junction between two neurons. At a synapse the terminal fibre of an **axon** reaches out to, but does not touch, the dendrite of the next neuron. The small gap between them is called the **synaptic cleft** or synaptic gap. When a neuron is stimulated a nerve impulse – the result of a change in electrical polarity across its membrane – travels at high speed along its axon. The tip of the axon terminal releases molecules of a chemical called a neurotransmitter, such as acetylcholine. This crosses the synaptic gap in a matter of milliseconds and depolarizes the membrane of the receiving dendrite, thereby generating a new impulse which passes along the second neuron. This is a one-way process that ensures nerve impulses travel only in one direction. Some association neurons in the brain form hundreds or thousands of synapses with other neurons.

Nucleus
Cell body
Myelin sheath
Axon
Schwann cell nucleus produces myelin
Nodes of Ranvier
Dendrite

▲ **Neuron** A neuron divides into three parts: a cell body that contains the cell's nucleus; short, branched processes called dendrites that receive nerve impulses from other neurons and carry them towards the cell body, and the axon, or nerve fibre, typically the longest part of the neuron – it can reach up to 1 m (3.3 ft) in parts of the PNS – which carries a nerve impulse to another neuron or a muscle. The axons of some neurons are insulated by a fatty myelin sheath which increases the speed of transmission of nerve impulses along the neuron to up to 350–400 kmh (200–250 mph).

▲ **TEM** of a synapse between two neurons. The triangular end of the axon of one neuron (yellow, upper centre) releases neurotransmitter across a synaptic cleft to the next neuron (lower right).

THE BRAIN

As the body's control centre, the brain receives input from inside and outside the body, correlates and stores incoming information, makes decisions and sends instructions. It automatically monitors and regulates body processes, controls movements and enables us to think, perceive and be self-aware. Protected within the skull, the brain is a soft organ weighing some 1.5 kg (3 lb). Within it are four connected cavities – ventricles – that produce cerebrospinal fluid, a constantly-moving clear liquid that acts as a shock absorber and delivers nutrients. Packed into the brain are more than 100 billion neurons. Making up just 2% of body's mass, it consumes 20% of the body's energy. It is divided into three main parts: the forebrain, cerebellum and brain stem.

Forebrain

The largest part of the brain, the forebrain deals with conscious actions, emotions and homeostasis. Its main structures are the cerebrum, limbic system and diencephalon (thalamus and hypothalamus).

Cerebrum

The cerebrum makes up 85% of the brain's weight. It is highly developed in humans and gives us our cognitive skills and generates consciousness, our sense of self-awareness. It is divided into left and right halves – hemispheres – linked by a 'bridge' of nerve fibres called the corpus callosum. Their surface is heavily folded by numerous gyri (ridges) and sulci (grooves) and each has four lobes:

Parietal lobe – perception of touch, pain and similar sensations

Frontal lobe – thought, emotions, speech, skilled movements

Temporal lobe – sound recognition and memory storage

Occipital lobe – interprets visual images.

The left hemisphere receives sensory input from, and controls the movement of, the right side of the body and is responsible for language, numbers, problem solving and logical behaviour, while the right hemisphere deals with the left side of the body, as well as art appreciation, music, facial recognition, imagination and insight. Each

The brain

Limbic system

Optic chiasma

Amygdala

Parietal lobe

Frontal lobe

Occipital lobe

Temporal lobe

Cerebral cortex – grey matter

White matter

Right hemisphere of cerebrum

Corpus callosum

Fornix

Thalamus

Hippocampus

Hypothalamus

Pituitary gland

Brain stem

Cerebellum

Spinal cord

hemisphere has three basic regions: cerebral cortex, white matter and basal nuclei.

• Cerebral cortex

This thin layer of grey matter around 4 mm (0.15 in) thick covers the outside of the cerebrum. The cortex processes and stores incoming information and makes possible thought, speech, creativity, perception, movement and all aspects of conscious behaviour. It consists of the cell bodies of billions of association neurons, each linked to hundreds or thousands of other neurons to create a communication network of unimaginable complexity. The extensive folding of the brain's surface greatly increases the amount of cerebral cortex that can fit inside the limited confines of the skull. Distinct areas of the cerebral cortex of each hemisphere carry out different tasks. These areas fall into three groups: motor areas trigger body movements; sensory areas receive input from skin, eyes, ears, tongue and nose and other sensors and association areas, which make up 75% of the cerebral cortex, interpret and analyse information and are involved in memory, learning and understanding.

• White matter and basal nuclei

White matter lies within the cerebral cortex and consists of the axons (nerve fibres) of association neurons. It provides the 'wiring' that links areas of the cerebral cortex and enables this 'higher centre' to communicate with other parts of the brain, and with other parts of the body by way of the brain stem, spinal cord and peripheral nerves. Basal nuclei are 'islands' of grey

matter within the white matter that help to regulate body movements. They work with the motor cortex, thalamus and cerebellum to plan, monitor and co-ordinate the contraction of skeletal muscles so that the body moves smoothly.

Limbic system

Sometimes called the 'emotional brain' the limbic system is a ring of structures including the amygdala (fear and anger), hippocampus (helps to establish memories) and fornix (links parts of the limbic system) on the inner border of each cerebral hemisphere. It is responsible for emotional and instinctive behaviour including fear, anger, elation, disappointment, sadness, pleasure and sexual feelings. It plays a key part in memory, interacts with the cerebral cortex to give conscious awareness of our feelings and works with the hypothalamus to generate sex drive and arousal.

Diencephalon

The central core of the forebrain, the diencephalon is surrounded by the cerebral hemispheres and contains the paired thalamus and hypothalamus.

• Thalamus

The thalamus is the 'gateway' to the cerebral cortex. It sorts and edits sensory input before passing it to the sensory cortex and liaises with the cerebellum and motor cortex to co-ordinate movement.

• Hypothalamus

The hypothalamus monitors and regulates conditions in the body as the prime mover in homeostasis. Its key roles include:

1) Controlling vital functions by sending out instructions through the autonomic nervous system (see pp. 44–45) to regulate, for example, heart rate, breathing rate and blood pressure

2) Regulating the endocrine system by controlling the release of hormones from the pituitary gland (see pp. 58–59)

3) Acting as a centre for emotional responses, biorhythms and sex drive, through its links with the limbic system

4) Regulating water balance and thirst

5) Regulating hunger and satiety

6) Maintaining a constant internal temperature of 37°C (98.6°F)

7) Regulating the sleep-wake cycle.

Lateral ventricles

Third ventricle

Fourth ventricle

THE BRAIN

Cerebellum

Making up some 11% of the brain's mass the cerebellum ('little brain') lies below the cerebral hemispheres' occipital lobes and behind the brain stem. Like the cerebrum, the cerebellum has two halves or hemispheres, each with a thin outer layer (cortex) of grey matter – the cell bodies of millions of neurons – inside which is white matter made up of their axons. The cerebellum co-ordinates movements and maintains the body's posture.

The cerebellum constantly receives updates from the cerebral motor cortex, brain stem, proprioceptors (stretch receptors in muscles, tendons and joints that 'report' on the state of muscle contraction), balance receptors in the inner ear and from the eyes. This enables it to determine how the body is moving and its position. It compares this information with the instructions from the motor cortex to muscles about movement and posture. The cerebellum issues instructions to correct and fine tune messages from the motor cortex and provide the timing and correct sequence of skeletal muscle contraction to produce smooth, co-ordinated movements and ensure that the body is positioned correctly. All this happens subconsciously. Without the cerebellum's intervention, body movements would be uncoordinated and jerky.

Brain stem

The body's 'autopilot', the brain stem controls processes essential for life, such as breathing and heartbeat and produces automatic, programmed behaviours essential for survival, such as the startle reflex. It has tracts of nerve fibres that link the cerebrum and cerebellum with the spinal cord, relaying information between the 'higher' brain centres and the rest of the body. Its reticular formation plays a major role in controlling consciousness to produce, with the hypothalamus, the daily pattern of wakefulness and sleep.

Each part of the brain stem is c.2.5 cm (1 in) long. They are, from inferior to superior:

• **The medulla oblongata**, or medulla, contains several motor centres. The cardiovascular centre controls the rate and force of heart contractions to meet the body's needs and regulates blood pressure. The respiratory centre (with the pneumotaxic centre in the pons) controls the rate and depth of breathing through a negative feedback system by which breathing rate changes according to carbon dioxide levels in the bloodstream. Other centres are responsible for vomiting, hiccupping, sneezing and coughing.

• **The pons** ('bridge') – the swollen middle section of the brain stem – relays information between the rest of the brain and the spinal cord. Certain fibres provide the link between the cerebral hemispheres and the cerebellum that lies dorsal to the pons.

• **The midbrain** lies at the top of the brain stem. A reflex centre that controls the subconscious movement of the eyes, head and neck in response to external visual stimuli, it produces the sudden turning of the head – the startle reflex – in response to sound stimuli. It is also involved in the 'fight or flight' response by linking the amygdala and autonomic nervous system.

▶ *MRI scan of a human brain seen in side view, with the brainstem area highlighted (blue). The brainstem connects the spinal cord with the upper cerebral regions of the brain.*

▶ **Memory** begins with sensation from the body passing to the cerebral cortex. As the information is relayed through the thalamus, it is also passed to the mamillary body and into the limbic system. The stimulus passes through the fornix to the hippocampus and then outwards into the diffuse area of the cingulate gyrus. If the memory of a similar stimulus is aroused, the cerebral cortex may be activated.

Cingulate gyrus

Brain areas

Fornix

Mamillary body

Hippocampus

From the senses

▶ **Movement** initiated in the motor cortex and immediately modified by the adjacent suppressor cortical area before direct transmission to the muscles. Each muscular movement is assessed and modified by the cerebellum in conjunction with the thalamus. An unconscious co-ordination of movement with position, balance and vision has to be made so that other muscles automatically adjust to give conscious movement.

Motor area

Suppressor area

Cerebellum

Thalamus

Pathways

Tracts

Spinal cord

▶ **Emotions** are a complex integration of conscious reaction, memory and instinctive desires. The frontal lobes and limbic systems both affect the hypothalamus, with its centres for anger, thirst, appetite and sexual desire. These may be stimulated to interact with the motor activity in the brain stem causing alterations in heart and respiratory rates and muscle tone. The hypothalamus also stimulates the pituitary gland.

Limbic system

Input

Pituitary gland

Hypothalamus

Heart and respiratory rates

Stem

To other organs

THE SPINAL CORD

Spinal cord

The spinal cord provides a vital communication link between the brain and the body by way of paired spinal nerves (spinal nerves are described in more detail on pp. 42–43) that arise from it, relaying information between body and brain. It also processes some incoming information, being involved in many reflex actions (see below). Linked to the brain by the brain stem, the spinal cord is a column of nervous tissue packed with millions of neurons. It has an average length of 45 cm (18 in) in adults, is no wider than a finger at its midpoint and extends down the back from the foramen magnum (the large opening in the base of the skull) to the level of the first lumbar vertebra. Just as the brain is protected by the skull, the delicate tissue within the spinal cord is protected by the vertebral foramina of consecutive vertebra which form a bony tunnel, called the **vertebral canal**, along which the spinal cord runs.

Internal structure

Approximately oval in section, the spinal cord can be divided internally into two clear zones. In its centre is a butterfly-shaped mass of **grey matter**. Grey matter contains the axon terminals of sensory neurons which carry nerve impulses from receptors to the spinal cord, the cell bodies of motor neurons which travel from the spinal cord to carry nerve impulses to muscles and glands and association neurons which relay nerve impulses between sensory and motor neurons. Surrounding the grey matter is a cylinder of **white matter**. This consists of nerve fibres, arranged in bundles called tracts, that relay messages between the brain and the peripheral nervous system. Ascending tracts (sensory) carry information about body sensation, which has arrived through sensory neurons in spinal nerves, to the brain; descending tracts (motor) carry instructions from the brain that then travel along the motor neurons in spinal nerves to the body's muscles and glands.

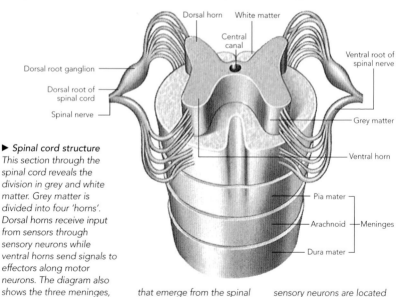

▶ *Spinal cord structure*
This section through the spinal cord reveals the division in grey and white matter. Grey matter is divided into four 'horns'. Dorsal horns receive input from sensors through sensory neurons while ventral horns send signals to effectors along motor neurons. The diagram also shows the three meninges, the membranes that surround and protect the spinal cord, and the two roots of each spinal nerve *that emerge from the spinal cord. The dorsal root contains sensory neurons which carry incoming nerve impulses – the cell bodies of* *sensory neurons are located in the dorsal root ganglion – while the ventral root contains motor neurons which carry outgoing signals.*

Meninges

Three cylinders of connective tissue, called the meninges, surround the spinal cord. On the outside is the **dura mater**, below which is the **arachnoid**, which, in turn, surrounds the **pia mater**. Circulating in the subarachnoid space – between the arachnoid and the pia mater – and in the spinal cord's central canal, is a colourless, watery liquid called **cerebrospinal fluid** (CSF). CSF has two roles: it acts as a shock absorber, cushioning the spinal cord from knocks and shocks, and it delivers nutrients from, and removes wastes to, the bloodstream.

Reflexes

Reflexes are automatic, involuntary, unchanging, split-second responses, many of which protect the body from hazards. A simple example is the withdrawal reflex by which we automatically pull away our hand when it touches a hot or sharp object. Other reflexes include blinking

Reflex action If a person touches something hot, sensory receptors in the skin generate nerve impulses that travel to the spinal cord along sensory neurons. In the spinal cord, messages are relayed by association neurons to motor neurons that transmit nerve impulses to the upper arm muscles, which withdraw the hand from the source of the heat before the person is consciously aware of it.

and swallowing. Many reflexes involve the spinal cord, since this provides the shortest, and fastest, pathway to a response. This short pathway is called a **reflex arc**. It typically involves a receptor responding to a stimulus by generating an impulse that travels along sensory neurons, association neurons, and motor neurons to a skeletal muscle. Only after the rapid, reflex action happens do nerve impulses arrive in the brain, making the person consciously aware of the stimulus, perhaps feeling pain or crying out.

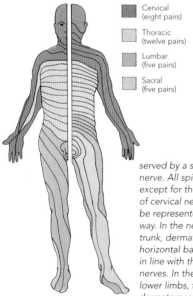

Cervical (eight pairs)

Thoracic (twelve pairs)

Lumbar (five pairs)

Sacral (five pairs)

▲ *Dermatomes A dermatome ('skin segment') is an area of skin that is*

served by a single spinal nerve. All spinal nerves, except for the first pair of cervical nerves, can be represented in this way. In the neck and trunk, dermatomes form horizontal bands that are in line with their respective nerves. In the upper and lower limbs, the dermatomes are aligned lengthways. Doctors can use a dermatome map to identify damaged nerves. A

lack of sensation in one particular skin area may enable the doctor to trace the problem back and identify the specific spinal nerve, possibly injured, that should normally serve this area. This dermatome map of the body divides up the skin's surface in terms of its innervation. Colour coding indicates whether a dermatome is served by cervical, thoracic, lumbar or sacral spinal nerves.

NERVES

These creamy white, glistening cords provide the information highways that arise from the central nervous system, or CNS (brain and spinal cord) and relay nerve impulses between the CNS and all regions of the body, including sense organs, muscles and glands. Each nerve consists of parallel bundles of hundreds or thousands of neurons or, more specifically, the long nerve fibres – or axons – of those neurons. The vast majority of nerves, called **mixed nerves**, carry a two-way traffic of nerve impulses because they contain the fibres of both motor and sensory neurons – purely sensory nerves or motor nerves are rare.

Inside a nerve, each bundle of neurons, or **fascicle**, is surrounded by a connective tissue sheath, the **perineurium**. Another connective tissue sheath, the **epineurium**, holds the fascicles together, along with their blood vessels. The epineurium protects the axons but permits bending of the nerve when the body moves. The largest, and longest, nerve, the **sciatic**, which supplies the leg, is about 2 cm (1 in) wide where it emerges from the lower part of the spinal cord. The thinnest nerves are no wider than a hair. Nerves are divided into two groups – spinal nerves and cranial nerves – according to which part of the CNS they arise from.

Spinal nerves

The 31 pairs of spinal nerves fan out in a repeating pattern from the spinal cord through openings between adjacent vertebrae called intervertebral foramina. All are mixed nerves. Their sensory neurons collect general sensory information from, for example, receptors in the skin relating to touch and pain, while their motor neurons carry instructions that control most of the body's skeletal muscles, as well as smooth muscles and glands. Spinal nerves divide into four groups (*see illustration, p. 41*): eight pairs of **cervical nerves** supply the neck, upper limbs and the diaphragm; twelve pairs of **thoracic nerves** supply muscles in the

Spinal nerves

Spinal cord

Dorsal root

Dorsal root ganglion

Ventral root

Intercostal nerve

Vertebra

Sympathetic ganglion chain of ANS (*see pp. 44–45*)

◄ *Spinal nerves This is a diagram of the thoracic region of the backbone and spinal cord. It shows how spinal nerves are formed by the merging of a dorsal root (carrying sensory nerve fibres) and a ventral root (carrying motor nerve fibres), both arising from the spinal cord. The dorsal root ganglion (pl. ganglia) is a swelling that contains the cell bodies of sensory neurons. The 12 intercostal nerves (the thoracic spinal nerves) supply the skin and muscles of the thorax and much of the abdominal wall.*

chest and back; five pairs of **lumbar nerves** supply the lower abdomen and parts of the lower limbs; five pairs of **sacral nerves** (and one pair of **coccygeal nerves**) supply reproductive organs and the bladder and other parts of the lower limbs. In the upper and lower parts of the spinal cord, spinal nerves merge to form an interconnecting nerve network called a **plexus**. The cervical plexus in the neck and the brachial plexus in the neck and axilla control the upper limbs; the lumbar plexus in the lower back and the sacral plexus in the pelvic region control the lower abdomen and lower limbs.

Nerve structure

Bundle of axons (nerve fibres)   Fascicle bound by perineurium

Cranial nerves

Twelve pairs of cranial nerves arise from the brain and emerge through foramina in the skull. The cranial nerves serve only the head and neck, apart from the **vagus nerves**, which extend into the thorax and abdomen. Most cranial nerves are mixed, carrying nerve impulses from sensors to the brain or carrying instructions from the brain to the muscles of the head and neck; three pairs, linked to special sense organs, are purely sensory. As well as being named, each pair of cranial nerves is also numbered using Roman numerals.

▲ *Coloured SEM of a section through bundles of nerve fibres (green). Each fibre consists of a nerve cell axon, the output process of a nerve cell, surrounded by a fatty insulating layer known as a myelin sheath. Myelin sheaths increase the transmission speed of the electrical nerve signals.*

▶ *Cranial nerves There are 12 nerves, I–XII (right), which arise from the under-surface of the brain. They supply the head, neck and major organs in the body. Sensory fibres are shown in blue, motor fibres in red. Three of them are solely sensory: olfactory I, optic II, and vestibulocochlear VIII. Two are mixed nerves, but are primarily motor in function: accessory XI to neck muscles, and hypoglossal XII to the tongue. Of the remaining mixed nerves: oculomotor III, trochlear IV* *and abducens VI supply the eye muscles; trigeminal V involves chewing and facial sensations; VII facial involves facial expression and taste in the anterior* *two-thirds of the tongue; glossopharyngeal IX involves swallowing and the remainder of taste and vagus X supplies chest and abdominal organs.*

43

AUTONOMIC NERVOUS SYSTEM

The autonomic nervous system (ANS) is the section of the nervous system that, second by second, automatically regulates involuntary functions – such as heart rate, digestion and pupil size – in order to help in the process of home-ostasis (maintaining a stable environment inside the body) and to enable the body to respond to the changing external and psychological demands on the body by causing arousal or quiescence.

How the ANS works

The ANS is a purely motor system with axons (nerve fibres) of motor neurons running from the central nervous system (CNS) to target structures: smooth (involuntary) muscles in the walls of body organs, such as the bladder, small intestine and blood vessels; glands, such as the adrenal and salivary glands, and the cardiac muscle in the heart. Changes in the internal and external environment are detected by sensors that send a constant stream of impulses along sensory neurons to the CNS, notably to centres in the brain stem which are, in turn, regulated by the hypothalamus, the ultimate controller of the ANS. Incoming information is processed in the CNS and signals are sent out along the motor neurons of the ANS to target organs.

Two divisions

The ANS has two divisions – sympathetic and parasympathetic – that have opposite effects. Target organs receive a supply of nerve fibres from both of them. The two antagonistic ANS divisions provide a self-regulating, dynamic balance that can be shifted, when necessary, to meet the body's demands. The **sympathetic division** is generally excitatory, prepares the body for stress and encourages energy expenditure. Sympathetic dominance increases heart rate and blood pressure, increases breathing rate, increases blood flow to the muscles, widens the pupils

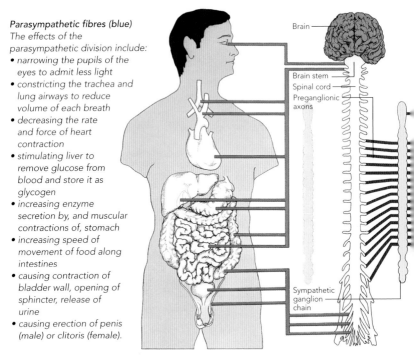

Parasympathetic fibres (blue)
The effects of the parasympathetic division include:

- *narrowing the pupils of the eyes to admit less light*
- *constricting the trachea and lung airways to reduce volume of each breath*
- *decreasing the rate and force of heart contraction*
- *stimulating liver to remove glucose from blood and store it as glycogen*
- *increasing enzyme secretion by, and muscular contractions of, stomach*
- *increasing speed of movement of food along intestines*
- *causing contraction of bladder wall, opening of sphincter, release of urine*
- *causing erection of penis (male) or clitoris (female).*

Brain

Brain stem
Spinal cord
Preganglionic axons

Sympathetic ganglion chain

and stimulates the liver to release energy-rich glucose into the blood. The sympathetic division also stimulates the adrenal glands to release adrenaline and noradrenaline, two hormones that mimic and prolong the effects of the sympathetic division. The **parasympathetic division** restores and conserves resources when the body is resting or recovering. Parasympathetic dominance produces calm and quiescence by slowing heart and respiratory rates and by prioritizing digestion in order to take in supplies of raw materials and energy and to store glucose in the liver ready for the next stressful episode.

Nerve fibres (axons) of the sympathetic division leave the thoracic and lumbar sections of the spinal cord through spinal nerves while nerve fibres of the parasympathetic division leave the brain stem through cranial nerves and the spinal cord through spinal nerves. Unlike the somatic nervous system – where single motor neurons run from the CNS to the target skeletal muscle – in the ANS two motor neurons runs in series, one following the other. The axon of the first neuron (called the **preganglionic axon**) runs from the CNS to a swelling called a **ganglion**, which contains a mass of axon terminals and acts as a relay station. The axon of the second neuron (**postganglionic axon**) runs from the ganglion to the target muscle or gland. In the sympathetic division, ganglia are linked in a vertical sympathetic chain, close to and on either side of the spinal cord. In the parasympathetic division, ganglia lie close to or within the target organ. The two divisions have opposite effects on target organs because their nerve endings release two different neurotransmitters which have an excitatory or inhibitory effect depending on the organ: sympathetic nerve endings release noradrenaline and parasympathetic nerve endings release acetylcholine.

Post-ganglionic axons

Sympathetic fibres (red)
Effects of the sympathetic division include:
- *widening the pupils to admit more light*
- *widening the trachea and lung airways to increase the volume of each breath*
- *increasing the rate and force of heart contraction*
- *decreasing enzyme secretion by, and muscular contractions of, stomach*
- *stimulating liver to release glucose into blood*
- *decreasing speed of movement of food along the intestines*
- *causing relaxation of bladder wall, closing of sphincter, thereby inhibiting release of urine*
- *causing ejaculation (male) and contraction of vagina (female)*

◀ *Autonomic Nervous System (ANS) The two divisions of the ANS spread out from both sides of the brain stem and/or spinal cord. For purposes of clarity, only half of each division is shown in this diagram. Some of the effects of the two divisions are described above.*

TOUCH AND PAIN

Without a constantly updated input of information about conditions inside or outside the body, it would be impossible for the brain to function. This information is provided by a range of sensory receptors. These detect stimuli – changes in their local environment – and generate nerve impulses which are transmitted along sensory neurons to the central nervous system (CNS) and then to the relevant sensory area of the brain. Many receptors, such as those for taste, smell, sight, hearing and balance – the five 'special senses' (described in detail on pp. 48–55) – are located in discrete sense organs (tongue, nose, eyes and ears) in the head. Touch, on the other hand, is known as a general sense because its receptors are scattered throughout the body.

Touch

Touch is a blanket term used to describe the sensations evoked by a range of receptors in the skin. The skin, as already described (see pp. 12–13), provides a large sensory interface between the body and its surroundings that enables humans to perceive a broad range of sensations including the chill of a dip in an icy sea, the pain of a paper cut, the softness of velvet or the pressure caused by holding a pen between finger and thumb. Perception, as with any sense, occurs when a person becomes aware of the sensation, following processing by the cerebral cortex of the 'raw' input of nerve impulses from the receptor.

Sensory receptors involved in touch differ according to the stimuli to which they respond. Mechano-receptors generate nerve impulses when they are pulled, pushed or squeezed. They are also found as **proprioceptors**, or stretch receptors, in muscles and tendons where they detect tension and send messages to the brain that enable it to maintain the body's posture. **Thermoreceptors** respond to cold or heat. **Nociceptors** respond to painful stimuli.

Receptors in the skin

The majority of sensory receptors in the skin are mechanoreceptors – their roles are related to their relative 'depth' in the dermis. **Merkel's discs**, which extend into the epidermis near to the skin's surface, detect light touch and pressure, helping to sense its source. **Meissner's corpuscles**, located just below the epidermal/dermal interface, also sense light touch. Deeper in the dermis, **Ruffini's corpuscles** respond to continuous touch on the skin. Deeper still, the larger **Pacinian corpuscles** detect vibration and firm, heavy pressure. All of these mechanoreceptors are encapsulated, that is enclosed, by a membrane. The remaining receptors are free nerve endings that detect movement of hairs (also mechanoreceptors), heat and cold and also pain.

Nerve impulses from skin receptors are carried by sensory neurons – via the spinal nerves, spinal cord, brain stem and thalamus – to the sensory area of the

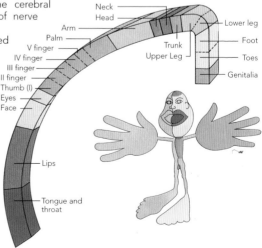

Neck
Head
Arm
Palm
V finger
IV finger
III finger
II finger
Thumb (I)
Eyes
Face
Lips
Tongue and throat

Lower leg
Foot
Trunk
Upper Leg
Toes
Genitalia

▶ *Homunculus This odd representation of the body, called a homunculus, shows the relative amount of brain power in the sensory cortex that is devoted to the variable numbers of sensory receptors in different parts of the body.*

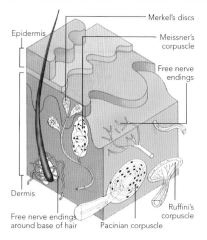

Epidermis

Merkel's discs

Meissner's corpuscle

Free nerve endings

Dermis

Ruffini's corpuscle

Free nerve endings around base of hair

Pacinian corpuscle

▲ *Skin receptors This section through the skin shows its two layers, the thinner protective epidermis and the thicker dermis. Most sensory receptors are located in the dermis, although some may extend into the epidermis.*

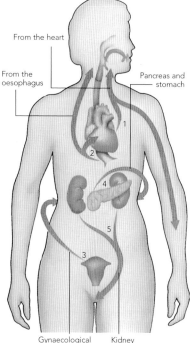

From the heart

From the oesophagus

Pancreas and stomach

1
2
4
5
3

Gynaecological   Kidney

cerebral cortex. Touch receptors are not evenly distributed over the skin. Some areas – such as the fingertips and lips – have many more receptors than others – such as the back – making them far more sensitive. This explains why blind people can use their fingers to 'read' Braille script. Because of this uneven distribution, a larger portion of the sensory cortex is needed to deal with sensory input from, say, the fingers than from the elbow.

Pain

Pain receptors, or **nociceptors**, are found not only in the skin but in most other parts of the body – including joints, the stomach and muscles – apart from the brain. They are stimulated by damage to tissues, typically by chemicals released by damaged cells, or by intense pressure or heat. Pain serves a useful purpose by alerting the body to actual or potential tissue damage. Somatic pain arises from skin, muscles and joints and can be either superficial – a sharp pain that can make someone cry out – or deep – an aching or burning feeling – that comes from muscles, joints or deep in the skin. Visceral pain (*see* referred pain below) is a dull ache or gnawing pain caused by the stretching or irritation of nociceptors in thoracic and abdominal organs.

◄ *Referred pain Internal organs and structures are well supplied with nerves, but pain is diffuse and poorly located compared with skin sensation (below). Most of the pain is produced by stretching and contracting, hence the pain of colic. Internal pain will cause stimulation of local nerves in a segment of the spinal cord: this makes it appear that the pain is coming from the skin which is supplied by the sensory nerves. The heart (1) and oesophagus (2) refer pain to the neck, shoulders and arms, the uterus (3) and pancreas (4) to the lumbar region and the kidneys (5) into the groin. Diaphragmatic pain may be referred to the shoulders, as the phrenic nerve of the diaphragm is formed from the spinal nerves in the neck, which also supply the shoulders.*

TASTE AND SMELL

Taste and smell are linked senses. First, they are located in close proximity to each other. Second, they complement each other and enable human beings to perceive flavours. Third, they both utilize the same type of sensory receptors, called **chemoreceptors**. These are sensors that detect dissolved chemicals. Those in the tongue respond to chemicals in food and drink; in the nose they respond to airborne chemicals. Chemoreceptors generate nerve impulses which travel to the brain.

Taste

The tongue is the organ of taste. This highly mobile, muscular organ moves food while it is being chewed and mixed with saliva, and also aids in the formation of words during speech. The tongue's surface is covered by tiny projections called **papillae**, which give it a characteristic bumpy appearance. There are three types of papillae: spiky **filiform papillae** cover the tongue and give its surface a rough texture to grip food during chewing and swallowing, mushroom-like **fungiform**

papillae are found near the edges and tip of the tongue and between seven and ten large **circumvallate** (or vallate) **papillae** form a V shape at the back of the tongue.

Housed in the sides of fungiform and circumvallate papillae are some 10,000 receptors called **taste buds**. Each consists of between 40 and 60 sensory and supporting cells arranged like the segments of an orange. Tiny 'hairs' (taste hairs), called **microvilli**, project from sensory cells into the opening of the taste bud, called the **taste pore**, on the side of the papilla. When food is chewed, its constituent chemicals, such as sugars, dissolve in saliva and flow into the taste pore and make contact with receptors on the taste hairs. These then generate nerve impulses that travel to the gustatory (taste) area of the cerebral cortex where tastes are perceived. Taste buds can detect just five tastes – sweet, sour, salt, bitter and umami (meaty) – but when combined with sensory data from the nose, the brain can distinguish between a wide range of flavours. The tongue also contains receptors for touch and pressure – allowing the texture

▼ **Tongue and taste buds** *This shows a detailed view of the surface of, and a section through, the tongue from a posterolateral view.*

Epiglottis

Lingual tonsil

Filiform papilla

Circumvallate papilla

Fungiform papilla

Taste bud

Salivary gland

of food to be determined – and for heat and cold – allowing the eater to distinguish between hot potatoes and ice cream. Pain receptors detect chemicals in spicy 'hot' food such as chillies.

Smell

Smell receptors are located in a postage-stamp sized area (c.2.5 sq cm/0.4 sq in) in the upper parts of the nasal cavity on either side of the basal septum. This area of olfactory epithelium contains around 10 million olfactory receptors, from which project between 6 and 20 hair-like cilia that detect odour molecules. When a person breathes in, air is carried high into the nasal cavity where the odour molecules it is carrying dissolve in watery mucus. Once dissolved, the odour molecules attach themselves to the cilia, which generate nerve impulses that are carried to the temporal lobe of the cerebral cortex (where they are perceived as smells), as well as to the limbic system, which, since this part of the brain deals with emotions and memories, explains why certain smells can evoke such power-

▼ *Olfactory receptors* This SEM shows cilia (coloured blue) projecting from an olfactory receptor in the nasal cavity.

ful memories. The sense of smell is 10,000 times more sensitive than taste, and can detect more than 10,000 different odours. There appears not to be 10,000 different receptor sites on the cilia of olfactory receptors. Instead, it seems that each smell is made up of one or more components from a set of 100 or so basic smells. It is to these basic smells that receptors respond.

Together, taste and smell allow humans to detect a range of flavours, which enhances, for instance, the enjoyment of a good meal. Of the two, smell is the 'senior' partner, as becomes clear when someone has a heavy cold and cannot discern any flavour at all. The perception of smells and/or tastes automatically causes the release of saliva from the salivary glands, and gastric juice from gastric glands, to aid in the process of digestion. Smell and taste also allow us to avoid harm by, for example, early detection of burning or being able to spit out food because it smells and tastes 'off'.

Olfactory nerves (I) passing through holes in cribriform plate of ethmoid bone

Olfactory bulb

Nasal cavity

Olfactory receptors

Hard palate

Tongue

Branches of VII and IX cranial nerves

▲ *Nerve pathways* This section through the head shows the routes taken by sensory fibres from olfactory and taste receptors to the brain. Nerve fibres of olfactory nerves (cranial nerve I) pass from olfactory receptors through tiny holes in the ethmoid bone (which forms the roof of the nasal cavity) and synapse with fibres in the olfactory bulb, an anterior extension of the brain. In the tongue, a branch of the facial nerve (cranial nerve VII) carries impulses from the anterior two-thirds of the tongue to the brain. A branch of the glossopharyngeal nerve (cranial nerve IX) carries impulses from the posterior third of the tongue to the brain.

EYES AND VISION

Vision is the body's most important sense. The organ that detects light, the eye, is one of the most complex in the body and the 125 million photoreceptors it contains – receptor cells that generate nerve impulses when stimulated by light – make up 70% of the sensory receptors in the body. Light entering the eye is focused on photoreceptors at the back of the eyeball, rather like a camera focusing light onto a film. Nerve impulses generated in the eyes are carried by optic nerves to the brain where they are processed so that we can perceive visual images.

The eyeball

Each eyeball is about 2.5 cm (1 in) in diameter. It is cushioned by pads of fat, and is located within, and protected by, a bony socket, or orbit, in the skull in such a way that only the anterior one-sixth of the eye is visible from the outside. The exposed front of the eye is protected from dust and excessive light by eyelashes and by the eyelids that open and close regularly during blinking and sweep tears across the eye's surface. Produced by

lacrimal glands located just above the eye, and released through tear ducts onto the eyeball's surface, tears wet the front of the eye, wash away dust particles and kill bacteria, before draining through two openings in the inner corner of the eye into the nasal cavity.

Eye structure

The simplest way to examine its structure is to look at the three layers from which the eyeball is made (see diagram below). The outer layer consists of the tough, slippery sclera, which covers most of the eyeball and forms the visible white of the eye, and the cornea, the clear domed region that allows light to enter the eye. The middle vascular layer, or uvea, consists, in much of the eyeball, of the choroid. This dark layer supplies the other layers with blood and because of its blackness prevents the internal reflection of light. Anteriorly it thickens to form the ciliary body, which contains a ring of muscle. Projecting inwards from the ciliary body are the suspensory ligaments that hold the transparent lens, made from fibres containing the proteins called crys-

Horizontal section through the eye

Suspensory ligament

Cornea

Iris

Pupil

Lens

Aqueous humour

Ciliary muscles

Conjunctiva

Sclera

Choroid

Retina

Fovea

Optic disc (blind spot)

Optic nerve

Vitreous humour

Extrinsic muscle

tallins, in place. The **ciliary muscles** adjust the shape of the lens to fine-focus light already partly focused by the cornea. The vascular layer projects inwards, anterior to the ciliary body, to form the **iris**. The iris contains melanin pigment which, depending on its concentration, gives the eye a colour ranging from pale blue to dark brown. The iris also contains smooth muscle fibres, arranged in radial and circular fashion. The fibres automatically regulate the size of the central opening or pupil to control the amount of light entering the eye (*see* below).

The inner layer of the eye, the **retina**, covers the choroid and extends anteriorly to cover the ciliary body. It consists of an array of photoreceptors called rods and cones (*see also* pp. 52–53), and the nerve fibres that carry nerve impulses generated by the photoreceptors to the brain. The 120 million **rods** work best in dim light and produce black-and-white images. The five million **cones** work best in bright light, detect colours and provide the greatest detail. Rods are dispersed throughout the retina, while cones are concentrated in the **fovea**, the central point of the retina directly behind the lens. Retinal nerve fibres leave the eyeball through the optic nerve. At its exit point, the **optic disc**, there are no photoreceptors. This 'blind spot', where no light is detected, leaves a visual gap that is 'filled' by the brain.

Either side of the lens, the eye divides into two unequal cavities. The larger and posterior cavity is filled with the jelly-like vitreous humour. The smaller and anterior cavity is filled with watery aqueous humour. Both under slight pressure, the humours serve to preserve the shape of the eyeball.

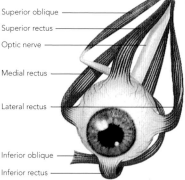

Superior oblique

Superior rectus

Optic nerve

Medial rectus

Lateral rectus

Inferior oblique

Inferior rectus

▲ **Pupil reflex** The retina is very sensitive to light. Too much light (**A**) distorts colour and is dazzling. The pupils vary in size and thus reduce or increase the amount of light entering the eye. Bright light causes a reflex nervous reaction, controlled by centres in the midbrain. The circular pupillary muscle (**1**) in both irises contracts and the radial fibres (**2**) extend, thus narrowing the diameter. Poor light (**B**) will make both pupils dilate, allowing sufficient light to stimulate the cells in the retina (**3**).

▲ **Eye muscles** The eyeball is moved by six extrinsic, or external, strap-like muscles. Movements of both eyes are co-ordinated by the brainstem so that they do not move independently in different directions. The superior rectus makes the eye look upwards. The inferior rectus makes the eye look downwards and inwards. The medial rectus makes the eye look medially. The lateral rectus makes the eye look laterally. The superior oblique swivels the eye so it looks downwards and outwards. The inferior oblique makes the eye look upwards and outwards.

EYES AND VISION

How the eye works

When light enters the eye from an object, it is refracted (bent) first by the cornea and then by the lens to produce an inverted, clearly focused image on the retina that will enable the brain to produce a clear view of the outside world. Fine adjustment to focusing is the role of the **lens** because, unlike the cornea, it has elasticity and can change shape in order to focus light from any object whether it is nearby or far in the distance. When looking at distant objects, the ring of **ciliary muscle** around the lens relaxes. The **vitreous humour** pushes outwards to increase the diameter of the ciliary body, causing the suspensory ligaments to pull on the lens and make it flatter, thereby providing the right shape to focus the nearly parallel light rays from the faraway object.

When looking at an object nearby, the ciliary muscle contracts, thereby reducing its diameter, the suspensory ligaments become less taut and the lens reverts to its natural, rounder shape in order to focus the divergent light rays arriving from the nearby object. Changing lens shape, known as **accommodation**, is controlled automatically by the brain. Shortsightedness, or **myopia**, is caused by light rays being focused in front of the retina; long-sightedness or **hypermetropia**, is caused by light rays being focused behind the retina. Both can be corrected by glasses or contact lenses.

Focused by cornea and lens, light falls on the photoreceptors in the retina. These contain a visual pigment that undergoes a change when hit by light, and causes the generation of a nerve

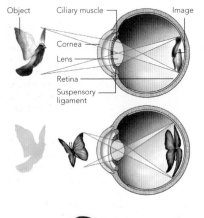

Object — Ciliary muscle — Image
Cornea
Lens
Retina
Suspensory ligament

◄ *Far and near*
These are the two images showing a section through the eyeball to reveal how the lens changes shape to focus light from far and near objects.

▲ **Colour blindness**
Ishihara test plate. Colour blind people will not be able to see the spade and fork.

▼ **Rods and cones** *This detailed view of the retina shows the arrangement of rods (blue) and cones (green), and their links to the nerve fibres which leave the eye through the optic nerve. It begins with the section through the eyeball showing light being focused on the fovea, with a zoom to a section through the retina and the detail of a rod and a cone.*

Retinal nerves
Retinal nerve fibres   Connecting neurons
Direction of light
Direction of nerve impulses
Cone
Rod

Field of vision – left eye
Binocular field of vision
Field of vision – right eye
Combined foveal image
Optic chiasma
Optic nerve
Optic tract
Lateral geniculate body
Left primary visual cortex
Right primary visual cortex

◀ *Visual pathways* Section though the eyes and brain to show the route taken by nerve impulses from the retina to the visual cortex.

cortex, and nerve impulses from the left half of each eyeball travel to the left primary visual area. They do so, on each side of the brain, along an optic tract which passes to the **lateral geniculate body**. This body relays nerve impulses to the primary visual areas, where movement and outlines are identified. Other cerebral areas refine the image so that it can be perceived. The slightly different inputs received from the left eye and the right eye enable the brain to construct a three-dimensional view of the world – its binocular field of vision – by combining the two inputs. This binocular, or stereoscopic, vision enables us to judge depth and distance accurately.

impulse which is transmitted to the visual cortex in the posterior region of the cerebral hemispheres. As already described (*see* pp. 50–51) there are two types of photoreceptors: rods and cones. **Cones** detect colours and provide the greatest detail and are concentrated mainly in the **fovea**, the point on which light falls when an object is looked at directly.

Visual pathways

Nerve impulses are carried away from the retina by nerve fibres that synapse with the photoreceptors. Because the eyes face forwards, they see the same view from slightly different angles, so the brain's visual processing area – the primary visual cortex – also receives slightly different sets of visual input. Nerve fibres travel along the optic nerves to a point of crossover called the **optic chiasma**. Here the nerve fibres partly cross over so that nerve impulses from the right half of each eyeball travel to the right primary visual

Colour blindness

Colour vision depends on the presence of three types of cones that each respond to a particular colour or wavelength of light: red, green or blue. About 10% of men and 1% of women (this is a sex-linked characteristic) have an inherited disorder called colour deficiency, or colour blindness, caused by the absence of one or more types of cone. This is commonly a red or green deficiency, resulting in an inability to distinguish between those two colours. A blue deficiency is rarer, as is total colour blindness. Defects in colour vision can be detected using Ishihara test plates (*see picture* opposite). The spade is purple and thus stimulates blue and green cones, and cannot be seen by the green colour blind. The fork is red so it is not seen by the red colour blind. Both are seen by those with normal colour vision.

HEARING

The ear is the organ of hearing and also plays a key role in the body's sense of balance. What most people refer to as the ear is, in fact, the outer flap, or pinna, that projects from the side of the head. The main part of the ear is concealed and protected within the temporal bone of the skull. The ear is divided into three distinct sections: the outer ear and middle ear, both of which are filled with air, and the fluid-filled inner ear.

Outer ear

The outer ear consists of the **pinna**, which is reinforced with elastic cartilage, and the 2.5 cm (1 in) long **auditory canal**. The outer ear serves to gather sound waves and direct them into the ear. Ceruminous glands in the skin lining the auditory canal produce a thick secretion called cerumen, or earwax, which, together with small hairs, keeps the canal clean and repels insects. Separating the outer and middle sections of the ear is a tightly stretched piece of skin called the **eardrum** or tympanic membrane.

Middle ear

Extending across the middle ear, from the **cochlea** to the oval window, are three tiny bones, or **ossicles**, named in Latin or

English for their shapes. The **malleus** (hammer) is attached to the eardrum; the **stapes** (stirrup) is attached to the oval window, the membrane-covered opening to the inner ear, and the central **incus** (anvil) connects the malleus and stapes through free-moving synovial joints.

Inner ear

Also called the labyrinth, the inner ear has two major parts. The **bony labyrinth** consists of channels and cavities that twist and turn through the temporal bone. These channels and cavities are filled with a liquid called **perilymph** and have three functional regions: the **cochlea**, which is involved in hearing, and the **vestibule and semicircular canals**, which are involved in balance (see below). The **membranous labyrinth** is a continuous series of membranous ducts that follows the contours of the bony labyrinth and floats in **perilymph**. The ducts themselves are filled with a fluid called **endolymph**.

The snail-shaped cochlea is divided by two membranes – the vestibular membrane and the basilar membrane – into three parallel channels: the **vestibular duct** runs from the oval window while the **tympanic duct** ends at the round window,

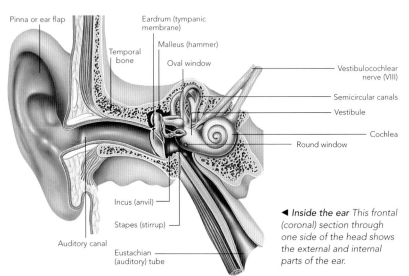

Pinna or ear flap

Eardrum (tympanic membrane)

Temporal bone

Malleus (hammer)

Oval window

Vestibulocochlear nerve (VIII)

Semicircular canals

Vestibule

Cochlea

Round window

Incus (anvil)

Stapes (stirrup)

Auditory canal

Eustachian (auditory) tube

◀ *Inside the ear This frontal (coronal) section through one side of the head shows the external and internal parts of the ear.*

a second membrane-covered opening between inner and middle ears and the **cochlear duct** lies centrally between the other two. Running along the cochlea is the spiral **organ of Corti**. This consists of about 15,000 mechanoreceptors, called hair cells, that 'sit' on the basilar membrane and from which project 'hairs' or microvilli that touch an overlying, roof-like membrane called the **tectorial membrane**. Nerve fibres from hair cells merge to form the cochlear branch of the vestibulocochlear nerve.

Hearing

Sound consists of waves of alternating high and low pressure that pass through the air and other media. Humans can detect sounds in the range 20 to 20,000 hertz (Hz), although this range decreases with age. The pinna directs sound waves into the outer ear, causing the eardrum to vibrate. As the eardrum vibrates, the three ossicles move, producing a piston-like action on the oval window as the base of the stapes is pulled

The cochlea Cut-away view of the cochlea (the arrows show the direction in which the sound waves travel).

Cochlear canal — Vestibular canal
Basilar membrane
Tympanic canal
Cochlear canal

Cochlear branch of vestibulocochlear nerve

Tectorial membrane
Organ of Corti

Vestibular membrane

Hair cells

Hairs embedded in overhanging tectorial membrane

Hair cells

Nerve fibres

Supporting cells

▲ *Balance* Ampullae (red) within the three semicircular canals detect movement of the head. Hair cells in the utricle and saccule (yellow) of the vestibule detect whether the head is upright or not. Input to the brain from all these structures enables it to detect the direction the body is moving, and its position relative to gravity. It is then able to control the body's balance and posture by sending instructions to its muscles.

in and out. This sets up vibrations in the fluid of the vestibular duct of the cochlea. The vibrations pass through the vestibular membrane, across the cochlear duct and set up vibrations in the basilar membrane. This causes the hair cells of the organ of Corti to move up and down, thereby distorting their hairs against the tectorial membrane. This bending generates nerve impulses that travel via the thalamus to the temporal lobe of the brain, where they are perceived as sounds. Vibrations returning along the tympanic duct are dissipated at the round window. High-pitched sounds are detected by hair cells near the oval window while low-pitched sounds are detected by hair cells nearer the tip of the cochlea. Loudness depends on the amplitude of the vibrations. The split-second difference in the time taken for sounds to arrive at the left and right ears gives the brain clues as to the direction of the sound.

ENDOCRINE GLANDS AND HORMONES

The nervous and endocrine (hormonal) systems combine to control and co-ordinate the body's activities. The nervous system uses high-speed electrical signals that stimulate muscles and glands: it acts rapidly with short-term effects. The endocrine system releases chemicals, known as hormones, that are carried by the blood and regulate the metabolic activities of cells thereby controlling processes such as growth, metabolism and reproduction. The endocrine system works more slowly and has longer-lasting effects. The two systems interact to control body activities.

Hormones

These chemical messengers are carried to all parts of the body by the bloodstream. Each affects specific target cells. Hormones are classified into one of two groups – amino-acid-based hormones and steroid hormones – according to their chemical structure. **Amino-acid-based hormones** – including amines, peptides, polypeptides and proteins – bind to specific receptors in the target cell membrane. This initiates chemical reactions that alter the target cell's metabolism. **Steroid hormones** – the hormones released by the ovaries, testes and the cortex of the adrenal glands – penetrate the target cell's membrane and interacts directly with genes in the nucleus to alter metabolism.

Endocrine glands

Endocrine glands, or ductless glands, release their secretions – hormones – into the bloodstream. The major endocrine glands are the pituitary, pineal, thyroid, parathyroid, thymus and adrenal glands. Other organs, including the testes, ovaries and pancreas, have significant areas of endocrine tissue and are also considered as endocrine organs. These organs, together with other areas of hormone-producing tissue, make up the endocrine system.

• Pituitary gland

The pituitary gland, the most important of the endocrine glands, releases nine or more hormones that either target other endocrine glands and stimulate them to release hormones or directly control body functions, such as growth. The hypothalamus controls the operation of the pituitary gland. A description of the structure and function of this gland is on pp. 58–59.

• Pineal gland

Hanging from the roof of the third ventricle in the posterior diencephalon, this tiny gland secretes ˙**melatonin**. Melatonin secretion follows a 24-hour cycle, with levels rising at night and falling around midday, in response to variations in light levels relayed to the pineal by the hypothalamus. High melatonin levels promote drowsiness and the hormone is believed to help set the body's 'internal clock'.

• Thyroid gland

Situated in the front of the neck below the larynx, the thyroid secretes three hormones. Thyroxine and triiodothyronine act on all body cells, increasing their metabolic rate and the pace of cell division. **Calcitonin** decreases levels of calcium in the blood by reducing the rate at which bone is broken down.

• Parathyroid glands

Embedded in the posterior part of the thyroid gland, the four tiny parathyroid glands secrete parathyroid hormone (PTH) which has the opposite effect to calcitonin because it increases the level of calcium in the blood by stimulating bone breakdown. Together, through negative feedback, PTH and calcitonin maintain stable levels of calcium in the blood.

• Thymus gland

Located posterior to the sternum, the thymus gland produces a number of hormones that are responsible for the normal development of T-lymphocytes and the immune response (see pp. 72–73). It is most active in children and shrinks throughout adulthood.

• Pancreas

Situated inferior and posterior to the stomach, the pancreas has an endocrine portion that releases two hormones – insulin and glucagon. **Insulin** reduces blood glucose levels by stimulating cells to take up glucose and the liver to store glucose as glycogen. **Glucagon** increases blood glucose levels by stimulating the liver to break down glycogen and release glucose into the bloodstream. Insulin and glucagon work together to maintain stable blood glucose levels.

• Adrenal glands

Sitting like 'hats' on top of the kidneys, the two adrenal glands divide into two parts. The **outer cortex** secretes steroid hormones called **corticosteroids**: gluco-corticoids help control cell metabolism and reduce stress and **mineralocorti-coids** control levels of sodium and potassium in the blood. The inner **adrenal medulla** secretes **noradrenaline** and **adrenaline** – two hormones that, untypically, work rapidly to help the body deal with stress, and produce the 'fight or flight' reaction.

• Ovaries and testes

As well as producing and releasing sex cells (ova and sperm), the ovaries and testes also release hormones – **oestrogen** and **progesterone** by the ovaries, and **testosterone** by the testes – that maintain secondary sexual characteristics and stimulate sex-cell production. Their roles are described in greater detail on pp. 98–101.

Regulating hormone levels

A process known as **negative feedback** controls hormone levels. If, for example, blood glucose levels rise, this stimulates release of insulin, but inhibits release of glucagon, from the pancreas, causing levels to fall. As glucose levels fall, this inhibits insulin release but stimulates glucagon release, causing glucose levels to rise.

Hypothalamus
Pituitary gland

Parathyroid gland
Thyroid gland

Thymus gland

Adrenal gland

Pancreas

Ovaries (in female)

Testis (in male)

◄ *Endocrine system*
This diagram shows the position of the body's main endocrine organs.

PITUITARY GLAND

The pituitary gland, or hypophysis, lies just below the brain, protected within the **sella turcica** of the sphenoid bone. Despite its relatively small size, the pituitary releases nine or more hormones, many of which trigger other endocrine glands to release hormones of their own. For that reason the pituitary gland is often referred to as the 'maestro of the endocrine orchestra' because it affects the activities of many other endocrine glands. It is, in fact, itself under the control of the **hypothalamus**, a part of the brain to which the pituitary is directly connected (see pp. 58–59). Together, the pituitary gland and the hypothalamus provide a direct link between the two co-ordinating and control systems of the body – the nervous and endocrine systems.

Structure of the pituitary gland

The pea-sized pituitary gland is attached to the hypothalamus superiorly by a stalk called the **infundibulum**. It consists of two lobes: one (anterior) glandular and the other (posterior) made of neural tissue. The **anterior lobe**, or adenohypophysis, makes up about 70% of the pituitary gland. It originates from the oral mucosa and is therefore composed of epithelial tissue. The hypothalamus gland communicates with the anterior lobe by way of the hypophyseal portal veins in the infundibulum. Neurons in the hypothalamus secrete release (and inhibiting) hormones, commonly polypeptides, that enter the **primary capillary plexus** in the superior infundibulum and are carried by the **hypophyseal portal veins** to the **secondary capillary plexus** in the anterior pituitary, where they regulate the secretion of hormones. Together the primary plexus, hypophyseal portal veins and secondary plexus form the **hypophyseal portal system** – a portal system is an arrangement of blood vessels where, unusually, capillaries merge to form veins which then branch into capillaries.

The **posterior lobe** (neurohypophysis) is part of the brain and is connected to the hypothalamus through a bundle of nerve fibres called the hypothalamic-hypophyseal tract, that runs through the infundibulum. The tract arises from neurons in the hypothalamus called neurosecretory cells. They make two hormones, known as neuro-hormones because of their mode of production, called

➡ Thyroid-stimulating hormone

➡ Growth hormone

➡ Prolactin

⇨ Follicle-stimulating hormone

➡ Luteinizing hormone

➡ Adrenocorticotropic hormone

Pituitary gland and hypothalamus (section)

antidiuretic hormone (ADH) and **oxytocin** – which are transported along nerve fibres to the posterior lobe. When hormones are required, the neurosecretory cells 'fire' and hormones are released from the axon terminals into blood capillaries in the posterior lobe and thence to their target tissues.

Anterior-lobe hormones

The anterior lobe of the pituitary gland synthesizes and releases its hormones in response to releasing hormones received from the hypothalamus. Two of the six anterior lobe hormones – **growth hormone** and **prolactin** – cause a direct effect on target organs; the other four – thyroid-stimulating hormone (TSH), adrenocorticotropic hormone (ACTH), follicle stimulating hormone (FSH) and luteinizing hormone (LH) – are referred to as **trophic hormones** because they regulate the action of other endocrine glands. The actions of these six hormones are now summarized.

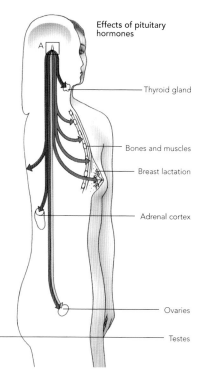

Effects of pituitary hormones

A

Thyroid gland

Bones and muscles

Breast lactation

Adrenal cortex

Ovaries

Testes

• **Growth hormone (GH)**
Also called somatotropin, GH targets body cells, especially those in bone and muscle and stimulates growth, in children, and repair by stimulating cell division.

• **Thyroid-stimulating hormone (TSH)**
Also called thyrotropin, TSH targets the thyroid gland and stimulates the release of two hormones, thyroxine and tri-iodothyronine, which, in turn, accelerate metabolic rate.

• **Adrenocorticotropic hormone (ACTH)**
ACTH targets the cortex (outer part) of the adrenal glands and stimulates the release of corticosteroid hormones that help regulate metabolism and play an important part in helping the body resist stress.

• **Follicle-stimulating hormone (FSH)**
In women, FSH targets the ovaries and stimulates maturation of an ovum and production of the sex hormone oestrogen. In men, FSH targets the testes and stimulates sperm production

• **Luteinizing hormone (LH)**
In women, LH targets the ovaries to trigger ovulation and stimulates the release production of the sex hormones oestrogen and progesterone. In men, LH (sometimes called interstitial cell-stimulating hormone or ICSH) stimulates production of the sex hormone testosterone.

• **Prolactin**
Prolactin targets the mammary glands in a women's breasts and stimulates milk production during and after pregnancy.

Posterior-lobe hormones

As described above, the posterior lobe receives its hormones from the hypothalamus. Both affect target organs directly, and their actions are outlined below.

• **Antidiuretic hormone (ADH)**
Also called vasopressin, ADH targets the kidneys and increases the amount of water returned to the blood during urine production, thereby reducing urine volume, conserving water and helping the body to maintain its water balance.

• **Oxytocin**
In women, oxytocin targets the uterus and stimulates muscle contraction at birth: it also stimulates the mammary glands to release milk during breastfeeding.

CIRCULATION

The circulatory or cardiovascular system consists of the blood vessels and the blood that is pumped along them by the heart. The circulatory system plays a vital role in maintaining homeostasis by controlling the concentration and composition of tissue fluid, by supplying cells with essential materials and removing their wastes, helping to keep the body warm and protecting the body against attack by pathogens. A vast network of blood vessels carries blood from the heart to the tissues and back to the heart once again in an unending circulation of this life-giving fluid.

Twin circulations

There are in fact two circulations within the cardiovascular system. These double, or twin, circulations consist of two loops that are linked by the two sides – left and right – of the heart, which acts as a double pump. The shorter of the two loops, the **pulmonary circulation**, carries oxygen-poor blood from the right ventricle of the heart to the lungs, where it picks up oxygen, and back to the left atrium of the

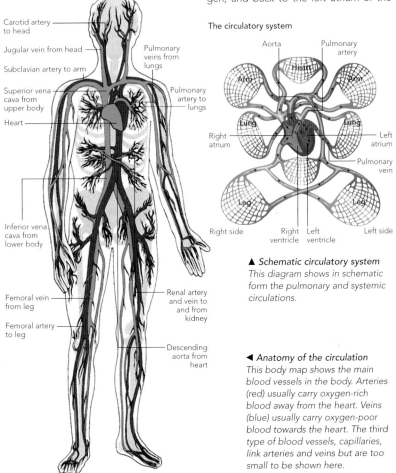

Anatomy of the circulation

Carotid artery to head

Jugular vein from head

Subclavian artery to arm

Superior vena cava from upper body

Heart

Inferior vena cava from lower body

Femoral vein from leg

Femoral artery to leg

Pulmonary veins from lungs

Pulmonary artery to lungs

Renal artery and vein to and from kidney

Descending aorta from heart

The circulatory system

Aorta

Pulmonary artery

Arm   Arm

Lung   Lung

Right atrium

Left atrium

Pulmonary vein

Leg   Leg

Right side   Right ventricle   Left ventricle   Left side

▲ Schematic circulatory system
This diagram shows in schematic form the pulmonary and systemic circulations.

◀ Anatomy of the circulation
This body map shows the main blood vessels in the body. Arteries (red) usually carry oxygen-rich blood away from the heart. Veins (blue) usually carry oxygen-poor blood towards the heart. The third type of blood vessels, capillaries, link arteries and veins but are too small to be shown here.

heart. The pulmonary artery, which carries blood to the lungs is unusual in being an artery that caries oxygen-poor blood: the pulmonary veins are similarly unusual because they are veins that carry oxygen-rich blood.

The longer loop, the **systemic circulation**, carries oxygen-rich blood from the heart to the rest of the body, and back to the heart. Oxygen-rich blood leaves the left ventricle of the heart and arrives through numerous branches in the tissues where it unloads oxygen and nutrients, and picks up metabolic wastes and returns along the veins to the right ventricle of the heart. Blood then re-enters the pulmonary circuit. A complete journey around the body takes about one minute.

Portal systems

Most veins carry blood back to the heart. However, in some cases veins carry blood from one organ to another. For example, the hepatic portal (or portal) vein carries food-rich blood from the capillaries of the small intestine to the capillaries of the liver, where the food is processed. A second vein, the hepatic vein, then collects venous blood from the liver and carries it towards the heart. This arrangement is called the hepatic portal system. The hypophyseal portal system carries releas-

▶ *The heart pumps blood around the body. The aorta (large red artery, upper left) carries blood to the body. To the left of the aorta is the upper part of the vena cava (blue). This vein carries oxygen-poor blood into the heart from the upper body. This blood then travels from the heart to the lungs (where it obtains oxygen) through the pulmonary artery (blue, centre) and returns to the heart through the pulmonary veins.*

ing hormones from the hypothalamus to the anterior lobe of the pituitary gland (*see* pp. 58–59).

The heart

This living pump contracts without a break to pump blood around the circulatory system. It consists mainly of cardiac muscle fibres that can contract of their own accord and without tiring. The heart has two halves – left and right – separated by a septum. The right side of the heart receives oxygen-poor blood from the body and pumps it along through the pulmonary circulation to the lungs, and then back to the left side of the heart. This pumps oxygen-rich blood through the systemic circulation to the body and then back to the right side of the heart once again. The internal structure of the heart and the mechanism of the heartbeat are described on pp. 62–63. Heart rate speeds up during exercise, and slows down when the body is at rest, because of the effects of the two branches of the autonomic nervous system on the pacemaker within the heart that controls its rate of contraction.

Blood pressure

When the lower chambers of the heart, the ventricles, contract, they exert a high pressure on the walls of the arteries that carry blood away from the heart. This pressure provides the driving force to push the blood around the body. As the ventricles relax before the next contraction, the blood pressure falls. The contraction is called systole, and the relaxation diastole. The higher (systolic) and lower (diastolic) pressures can be measured using instrument call mo-
m
p
b
t
is
her blood
neither too high

61

Position
The heart lies in the thorax behind the sternum and in front of the descending aorta and oesophagus. It rests on the central ligament of the diaphragm muscle. On either side are the two lungs. Above are the main blood vessels and the bifurcation of the trachea into the two main bronchi.

Basic facts
The heart weighs about 300 g (11 oz) and is about the size of a grapefruit. It has two atria, two ventricles and four valves. It receives blood from the two venae cavae and four pulmonary veins and expels it into the aorta and pulmonary artery. It pumps 7,200 l (12,670 pt) of blood a day at a rate varying between 60 and 160 beats a minute.

Anatomy
The heart is surrounded by the fibrous pericardium, containing the serous peri-cardial sac holding a small amount of fluid that allows frictionless movement. It consists of two pairs of chambers – atrium and ventricle – that act as separate pumps. The right side pumps deoxy-genated blood through the lungs – the **pulmonary circulation**. The left side pumps oxygenated blood from the lungs – the **systemic circulation**.

Atria and ventricles
The blood from the superior and inferior venae cavae enters the right atrium. The four pulmonary veins take blood to the left atrium.

The atrioventricular valves, tricuspid in the right and mitral in the left, have special muscles (the papillary muscles) and fine tendons (chordae tendineae) attached to the edges of the valve cusps to prevent them rupturing back into the atria during ventricular systole.

The left ventricle has thicker muscle than the right to sustain a higher systemic

The heart

- Aorta
- Superior vena cava
- Pulmonary artery
- Pulmonary veins
- Pulmonary valve
- Atria
- Aortic valve
- Mitral valve
- Chordae tendineae
- Tricuspid valve
- Papillary muscle
- Ventricles
- Inferior vena cava

Electrical system

- Sino-atrial node
- Atrioventricular node
- Bundle of His

Coronary circulation

- Right coronary artery
- Aorta
- Left coronary artery
- Coronary vein

blood pressure. The ventricles are closed by the aortic and pulmonary valves.

The heart is lined with endocardium, and divided by the interatrial and interventricular septa, while the remnants of the fetal circulation can be seen in the fibrous band of the ductus arteriosus.

The electrical system

To keep the heart beating, the sino-atrial node (or 'pacemaker') in the right atrium sends impulses through the two atria, causing atrial systole. It then stimulates the atrioventricular node to pass impulses rapidly down the bundle of His to cause ventricular systole (*see image* opposite, top right).

Coronary circulation

The myocardium has its own blood supply (*bottom left*) from the left and right coronary arteries – the first branches of the aorta – supplying different areas of muscle with a few anastomoses between them. The coronary (cardiac) veins drain venous blood into the right atrium.

▶ *A heartbeat In atrial diastole (**A**) blood flows from the inferior and superior venae cavae into the right atrium (**1**) and from the four pulmonary veins into the left atrium (**2**). The flow is increased during inspiration as the negative intrathoracic pressure also 'sucks' blood into the heart as well as air into the lungs. This results in sinus arrhythmia.*

*When ventricular systole ceases (**B**), the intraventricular pressure drops and the two atrioventricular valves – the tricuspid (**3**) and the mitral (**4**) – float open and blood starts to flow from the atria (**1**, **2**) into the ventricles. The sino-atrial node then initiates atrial systole and the blood is pumped past the valves, which are fully open, into the dilated ventricles.*

*Atrial systole ceases (**C**) when the electrical impulse reaches the atrioventricular node and passes down the bundle of His to start ventricular systole. Once atrioventricular valves (**3**, **4**) snap closed, the chordae tendineae and papillary muscles prevent them*

*bursting back into the atria. Venous blood can again flow into the atria (**1**, **2**), during atrial diastole and ventricular systole.*

*The rapidly increasing ventricular pressure (**D**) throws open the aortic (**5**) and pulmonary (**6**) valves with blood streaming into*

*the systemic and pulmonary circulations. The elasticity of the arterial walls causes the valves (**5**, **6**) to snap closed at the end of ventricular systole. The 'snap' of the opening and closing heart valves can be heard as 'lub-dub' through the chest wall.*

BLOOD

Pumped by the heart, blood flows along blood vessels, supplying the body's trillions of cells with all their needs, while ensuring that they are kept in stable surroundings. Blood makes up about 8% of an adult's mass, with 4 to 5 l (7 to 9 pt) of blood in a woman and 5 to 6 l (9 to 10.5 pt) of blood in a man. Blood is a connective tissue: its red blood cells, white blood cells and platelets are suspended in its liquid matrix, which is called plasma.

Functions of blood

Blood underpins homeostasis by helping to maintain a stable internal environment inside the body. The homeostatic functions of blood can be divided into three basic types: transport, regulation and protection. Blood **transports** oxygen from the lungs to all body cells, and glucose, amino acids and other nutrients from the small intestine. It removes metabolic wastes, such as carbon dioxide from all body cells and urea from the liver, and carries them to a point of elimination from the body, respectively the lungs and the kidneys. Blood helps **regulate** the body's internal environment by maintaining a constant pH in both blood and tissue fluid and by helping to maintain a constant body temperature by distributing heat from sources of production, such as the liver and muscles, around the body. Blood **protects** the body by preventing leakage from damaged blood vessels through blood clotting and by carrying white blood cells to sites of infection where they destroy invading pathogens.

Plasma

Yellow plasma is 90% water, 7% plasma proteins and 3% dissolved small molecules. Dissolved plasma proteins include albumin, which helps to maintain normal blood volume; alpha and beta globulins, which help transport some lipids and hormones; gamma globulins, or antibodies, which defend the body against infection; fibrinogen and other proteins involved in clotting and certain antibacterial proteins and metabolic enzymes. Other solutes include glucose, amino acids, fatty acids and other nutrients, carbon dioxide and nitrogenous waste products, hormones and sodium, potassium and other ions that help to maintain the normal concentration and pH level of the blood.

▶ *Blood composition*
If blood is spun in a centrifuge tube, its main constituents separate and their relative volumes can be estimated visually. The heaviest components – red blood cells – sink to the bottom of the tube while the lightest – plasma – remains at the top. White blood cells and platelets form a thin layer in between. Plasma makes up about 55% of the total volume, red blood cells about 44% and white cells and platelets about 1%.

Plasma

White cells and platelets

Red blood cells

Neutrophils in immature to mature form

Small and large lymphocyte

Monocyte

Platelets

Red blood cells

▲ *Blood cells This illustration shows many of the different types of blood cells (magnified). The three main types of white blood cells are neutrophils, lymphocytes and monocytes. Platelets are vital clotting agents. Red blood cells are the most numerous.*

Red blood cells

Erythrocytes (red blood cells) make up c.99% of blood cells, with some 5 million cells per cu mm (0.00035 fl oz) of blood, outnumbering white blood cells by 800 to one. Their function is to supply oxygen to all body cells. Each red blood cell is a flattened disc with a dimpled centre, giving it a biconcave profile. This shape provides a large surface area, relative to the cell's volume, for taking up and releasing oxygen. Red blood cells are also small – at c.0.007 mm (0.0003 in), just narrower than the diameter of the smallest capillaries – and have a natural elasticity, which enables them to squeeze along narrow capillaries in single file. Red blood cells lack a nucleus; instead they are packed with the protein **haemoglobin**, which gives them their red colour. As red blood cells pass through the lungs, where oxygen concentration is high, haemoglobin picks up oxygen to form oxyhaemoglobin; when red blood cells pass through the tissues, where oxygen levels are low because of its constant consumption by cells in cell respiration, oxyhaemoglobin unloads its oxygen and becomes haemoglobin. Oxyhaemoglobin gives arterial blood its bright red colour, while haemoglobin gives venous blood its dark red colour.

White blood cells

Although there are far fewer white blood cells than red blood cells – about 7,000 per cu mm (0.00035 fl oz) of blood – they play a vital role in defending the body against infection by pathogens. White blood cells have the ability to squeeze through capillary walls, by a process known as **diapedesis**, and enter the tissues. White blood cells are divided into three groups: granulocytes, monocytes and lymphocytes. **Granulocytes** are first on the scene if pathogens enter the body or if tissue is damaged. The commonest types, called **neutrophils**, are active phagocytes: they detect, surround, engulf and digest pathogens and debris. **Monocytes** are also phagocytic: in the tissues they become large, voracious hunters called **macrophages**. **Lymphocytes** play a key part in the immune response and are described in more detail on pp. 72–73.

Platelets

Platelets are cell fragments that lack a nucleus. They are about one-third the size of red blood cells, and are described in more detail on pp. 66–67.

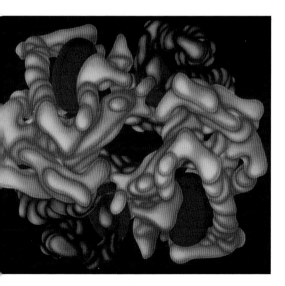

◀ *Haemoglobin This computer-generated model shows the structure of a haemoglobin molecule. It consists of four sub-units. Each subunit consists of a polypeptide chain (there are two pairs – blue or orange) and a haem molecule (red disc), a red pigment that contains at its core an iron atom. Each haem group can bind one oxygen molecule, so with 250 million molecules packed into a single red blood cell, that cell can carry about one billion oxygen molecules when fully loaded.*

Blood cell formation

Blood cells are produced, in adults, by red bone marrow located within the spongy bone found in the flat bones of the skeleton – skull, collar bones, shoulder blades, sternum, ribs, vertebrae and hip bones – and in the epiphyses of the femur and humerus. The cells that divide to produce blood cells are **stem cells** called haemocytoblasts. Their derivatives differentiate to form either red blood cells, granulocytes (neutrophils, eosinophils or basophils), agranulocytes or platelets.

While granulocytes continue to mature in bone marrow, the precursors of monocytes and lymphocytes move to the lymph nodes, spleen and other organs of the lymphatic system and continue their development there.

Red blood cells are produced, by a process called **erythropoiesis** at the rate of about 2 million per second. They have a life span of about 120 days, at which point they are worn out and need replacing. Old red blood cells are processed in the spleen and liver and their iron content

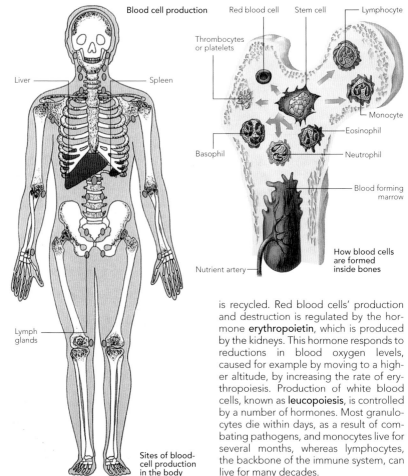

Blood cell production

Liver

Spleen

Lymph glands

Sites of blood-cell production in the body

Thrombocytes or platelets

Red blood cell

Stem cell

Lymphocyte

Monocyte

Eosinophil

Neutrophil

Basophil

Blood forming marrow

Nutrient artery

How blood cells are formed inside bones

is recycled. Red blood cells' production and destruction is regulated by the hormone **erythropoietin**, which is produced by the kidneys. This hormone responds to reductions in blood oxygen levels, caused for example by moving to a higher altitude, by increasing the rate of erythropoiesis. Production of white blood cells, known as **leucopoiesis**, is controlled by a number of hormones. Most granulocytes die within days, as a result of combating pathogens, and monocytes live for several months, whereas lymphocytes, the backbone of the immune system, can live for many decades.

Blood clotting

Blood clotting prevents excessive blood loss from a wound. Normally, circulating blood contains red cells, platelets, plasma, clotting factors and fibrinogen. Tissue-clotting factors lie trapped within cells surrounding each blood vessel (**A**). When damage occurs blood escapes from the broken vessel. Platelets congregate at the site and help to plug the wound. Tissue-clotting factors are released (**B**). The reaction of the platelets with plasma and tissue-clotting factors converts the soluble fibrinogen into insoluble threads of fibrin. The fibrin forms a mesh across the break (**C**). Platelets and blood cells become trapped in the mesh. The jelly-like mass shrinks and serum oozes out, leaving a clot (**D**). The clot dries out to form a scab under which the damaged tissue repairs itself.

Blood clotting

Blood groups

Although the red cells in different people look the same they are, in fact, dissimilar. They can be divided into four main groups, A, B, AB and O (*below*). The surface of the cells in each group is different and will act as an antigen to plasma from another group, which carries the antibody. This causes the cells to stick to each other by the process of agglutination. An individual with Group A cells will carry the antibody B in his plasma, those in group AB do not carry either antibody, while those in group O have both antibodies but the cells do not have either antigen. Thus blood from any group can be transferred into those of group AB, as they do not carry antibodies; group AB individuals are known as 'universal recipients'. Group O recipients can only receive blood from another group O donor, but can give blood to anyone and thus are known as 'universal donors'.

Antibodies in the plasma of the donor blood are quickly diluted by the recipient and the concentration is therefore too low to cause agglutination. The two commonest groups in western Europe are Groups A and O, each found in about 45% of the population, group B in about 10% and group AB is found in less than 5%.

The antigen-antibody reaction causes not only agglutination but also haemolysis – the breakdown of the red blood cells releasing haemoglobin into the circulation. This is an 'incompatible transfusion reaction' and can lead to fever, jaundice, kidney failure from blocking of the tubules with haemoglobin and even, in some cases, death.

▶ *Blood group compatability*
This chart shows blood group compatability between donor and recipient. Where the red blood cell symbol is smooth, there is compatability, where the symbol is rough, there is incompatibility. So, for example, a group O donor can donate blood to any other group, but can only receive blood from another group O person.

Laid end to end, the blood vessels of the body would stretch more than 150,000 km (93,000 mi). The three main types of blood vessels – arteries, veins and capillaries – are living, flexible structures that maintain blood flow in one direction, respond to the body's changing demands by diverting blood flow to particular areas and, in the case of capillaries, are 'leaky' enough to allow the outflow and inflow of fluid to deliver materials to, and collect them from, the body's cells.

Apart from capillaries, blood vessels share the same structure (*see* below) with four distinct layers or tunics – **endothelium** which allows the smooth flow of blood, **connective tissue**, **smooth muscle** and elastic fibres to confer strength and flexibility and a tough outer coat of **collagen** fibres – surrounding the central lumen. The three types of blood vessels differ in their lengths and diameters and the relative thickness of their walls.

Arteries

Arteries are elastic, thick-walled vessels that carry blood under high pressure away from the heart. All carry oxygen-rich blood, apart from the pulmonary trunk (artery) which carries oxygen-poor blood from the right ventricle to the lungs. The largest artery, the **aorta**, is about 2.5 cm (1 in) in diameter and carries oxygen-rich blood out of the left ventricle. Arteries branch repeatedly as they get farther away from the heart, giving rise to progressively smaller vessels. **Elastic arteries** are closest to the heart and include the aorta. When blood passes along them, their highly elastic walls first expand and then recoil – an action that smoothes out the dramatic pressure changes that occur when the heart contracts and then relaxes. The pressure wave passing along an elastic artery is called a pulse and can be felt at various points in the body, such as the wrist. **Muscular arteries** are smaller branches of elastic arteries. Contractions of the smooth muscle fibres in the walls of muscular arteries, under instructions from the autonomic nervous system, control the flow of blood along them. The smallest muscular arteries divide to form arterioles, vessels less than 0.3 mm (0.01 in) in diameter. These divide to form capillaries.

Artery

Vein

Both arteries and veins are tubes made of four layers:

Protective fibrous covering

Smooth muscle and elastic fibres

Connective tissue

Endothelial layer of cells

◄ *Comparing arteries and veins* The arteries carry blood away from the heart and the veins return it. Both arteries and veins (see opposite) are made in the same way with four layers: a protective fibrous coat, a middle layer of smooth muscle and elastic tissue that is thickest in the largest arteries, a thin layer of connective tissue and a smooth layer of cells – the endothelium.

Capillaries

The smallest blood vessels, having a lumen of 0.008–0.01 mm (0.0003–0.004 in) in diameter, capillaries nonetheless make up some 90% of the length of the blood vessel network. Their role is to get blood to all tissue cells. The capillary wall is just one cell thick and is leaky. Fluid, but not cells, from the blood passes out through the wall and into the tissue fluid that bathes tissue cells. This is how oxygen, food, etc. are transferred from blood to cells. As the capillaries weave their way through the tissues in capillary beds, the osmotic pressure of the blood increases, and this draws fluid containing wastes and secretions from cells back into the blood. Capillaries then merge to form **venules**, the smallest vein branches.

Veins

Veins carry blood from the tissues back to the heart. All carry oxygen-poor blood, except for the pulmonary vein which carries oxygen-rich blood from the lungs to the left atrium of the heart. The venules unite to form larger veins that finally empty into the inferior vena cava (lower body) and superior vena cava (upper body) that drain into the right atrium of the heart. Veins have thinner walls than arteries, as the blood that passes though them is under much lower pressure. (*See* venous blood flow below.)

▲ *This scanning electron micrograph (SEM)* image shows red blood cells (erythrocytes) passing from a capillary to a vein.

Veins and venous blood flow
The blood reaches the venous system through minute capillary vessels. It is through the capillary wall that oxygen and carbon dioxide, food and metabolites are exchanged with the interstitial fluid. Most of the interstitial fluid returns to the venous system, but some is collected by the lymphatic vessels.
The returning venous blood moves slowly due to low pressure and the veins can collapse or expand to accommodate variations in blood flow (right). Movement relies on the surrounding muscles, which contract (1) and compress the vein. Pulsation of adjacent arteries (2) has a regular pumping effect.

Semilunar valves (3) are found at regular intervals throughout the larger veins and these allow the blood to move only in one direction. They are more common in the legs. The veins frequently anastomose with each other so that the blood flow can

alter direction if there is any constriction or pressure from movement of muscles or ligaments.

LYMPH AND LYMPH ORGANS

In addition to the cardiovascular system, the body has a second, less familiar transport system – the lymphatic system. It consists of a network of blind-ending tubes, called lymphatic, or lymph, vessels and a number of associated lymphatic organs. The lymphatic system has two main functions: the transport of a fluid called lymph and the provision of sites for the cells of the immune system (see pp. 72–73) to attack and destroy invading pathogens.

Lymph

The lymphatic system plays a vital role in maintaining the normal volume of the blood. Every 24 hours some 24 l (42 pt) of fluid passes through the walls of blood capillaries to supply food and oxygen to tissue cells. It then removes carbon dioxide and other materials and returns through the capillary walls into the blood. However, some 3 to 4 l (5 to 7 pt) of fluid does not return in this way, and would accumulate in the tissues if it were not collected by fine, blind-ending lymph capillaries. These tiny vessels have tiny flaps that act like one-way swing doors and allow fluid into the lymph capillaries but not back into the tissues. The watery fluid, now called lymph, is returned by the lymph vessels to the bloodstream in order to ensure that its volume remains unchanged.

Lymph vessels

Reaching nearly every part of the body, lymph vessels form a one-way network of channels. Fine lymph capillaries permeate the tissues, where they collect lymph. They join to form larger vessels, called lymph-collecting vessels, that merge to form larger vessels called lymph trunks. The latter empty into the two largest lymph vessels, the thoracic duct and right lymphatic duct, that empty lymph into, respectively, the left subclavian vein and right subclavian vein and thereby back into the bloodstream. This completes the journey made by the fluid 'left behind' in the tissues back to the bloodstream. The lymphatic system has no equivalent of the heart to push lymph along. Instead

Right lymphatic duct

Left subclavian vein

Thoracic duct

Lymph node

Lymph trunk

Lymph vessel

◄ *Lymph vessels* This diagram shows how the network of lymph vessels joins up to form the two lymphatic ducts, which empty lymph into the bloodstream.

Incoming lymph vessel

Valve

Outgoing lymph vessel

Meshwork of reticular fibres

Germinal centre where lymphocytes multiply

▲ *Lymph node* This section though a lymph node shows the direction of lymph flow, and the meshwork of fibres that support macrophages and lymphocytes.

Spleen *Situated to the left of the stomach, and served by the splenic artery and vein, the spleen is the largest of the lymph organs. It has two main roles. First, it removes ageing red blood cells from the blood and salvages their iron for later use. Second, its macrophages remove pathogens and* *cell debris from the blood flowing though its sinuses (blood spaces), while lymphocytes initiate the immune response. White pulp consists of fibres that carry lymphocytes, while red pulp consists of blood sinuses and areas of connective tissue that are rich in macrophages.*

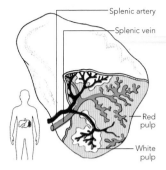

Splenic artery

Splenic vein

Red pulp

White pulp

this function is achieved by the skeletal muscles that surround lymph vessels and push lymph along them when they contract. Like veins, lymph vessels also have valves that prevent the backflow of lymph.

Lymph organs

Lymph (or lymphoid) organs including lymph nodes, the spleen (*see* above) and tonsils, form the part of the lymphatic system that defends the body by destroying pathogens and cancer cells. They contain lymphocytes and macrophages, white blood cells that that form a vital part of the immune system.

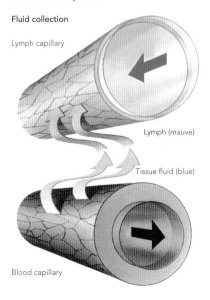

Fluid collection

Lymph capillary

Lymph (mauve)

Tissue fluid (blue)

Blood capillary

• **Lymph nodes**

These small bean-shaped swellings, each between 1 and 20 mm (0.04–0.8 in) in diameter, occur along lymph vessels. The lymph that passes through them contains not just clear tissue fluid but also bacteria and other pathogens, cell debris and possibly cancer cells. Inside a lymph node is a mesh of fibres that carries large numbers of macrophages and lymphocytes. Lymph nodes also produce large numbers of lymphocytes, up to 10 billion per day. As lymph passes though the lymph node, macrophages and lymphocytes detect and destroy pathogens and cancer cells and engulf any cell debris. The 'filtered' lymph then continues on its way back to the bloodstream. During certain infections the lymph nodes become inflamed and tender, a condition known as 'swollen glands'.

• **Tonsils**

Two tonsils at the back of the tongue, two at the back of the mouth and one in the upper throat form a ring of lymph tissue that protects the entrance to both digestive and respiratory systems. Lying in the mucosa, each tonsil contains blind-ending crypts that contain lymphocytes. These destroy bacteria, carried into the body by food or air, that migrate into the crypts.

• **Peyer's patches**

These are small patches of lymph tissue found in the wall of the lower small intestine and the appendix. They contain macrophages and lymphocytes that prevent the bacteria that are commonplace in the intestines from entering the human bloodstream.

DEFENCES AGAINST INFECTION

Every second, the body is exposed to a range of pathogens – including bacteria, viruses, protists and fungi – that can, if they enter the body's tissues and bloodstream, multiply and destabilize the body's normal homeostasis and thereby cause infections that may be fatal. Non-specific defences repel and attack any pathogens, while the specific defences – the immune system – destroy specific pathogens and retain a memory of them.

Non-specific defences

These are built into the body from birth and provide two lines of defence: surface barriers and defensive cells and chemicals.

Barriers and secretions

Surface barriers provide the first line of defence against pathogens and include the tightly packed cells of the skin and those of the mucous membrane lining the digestive, respiratory, urinary and reproductive systems. Secretions include **mucus** secreted by the mucous membranes of the nasal cavity, trachea and

▲ *Phagocytosis This SEM shows a phagocyte engulfing a pathogen. The phagocyte recognizes the bacterium, or other pathogen, by the chemical signals it sends out. It wraps itself around and engulfs the pathogen. The pathogen is taken into the phagocyte and digested. Neutrophils are often destroyed by this and form a mass of white liquid called pus at the site of infection. The process of binding phagocyte to pathogen is made more effective by coating the pathogen with complement.*

bronchi. Mucus traps pathogens, is carried to the throat, swallowed and digested by acidic gastric juice in the stomach. **Gastric juice** destroys bacteria entering the body in food or drink. Tears contain antibacterial lysozyme which kills bacteria as the tears flow over the eye.

Cellular and chemical defences

Should pathogens penetrate epithelial barriers and invade the tissues, a second line of non-specific defences involving defensive cells and chemicals swings into action.

• Phagocytes

Phagocytes, or 'cell eaters', are white blood cells (*see* pp. 64–65) that are attracted to sites of infection or damage and include neutrophils and macrophages that trap and engulf prey by phagocytosis (*see image*, below left).

• Natural killer (NK) cells

Found in lymph nodes and circulating in the blood, NK cells target cells infected by viruses as well as cancer cells. NK cells bind to these rogue cells and destroy them with toxic chemicals.

• Inflammation

When tissue damage occurs, local and white blood cells release chemicals including histamines that send out an alarm signal, making local blood vessels wider and more leaky, bringing in extra phagocytes and antibodies to fight infection. Increased blood flow also makes the area warm, swollen and tender, resulting in inflammation.

• Antimicrobial proteins

Two main groups of specific defence proteins are produced. **Interferon** is released by cells already infected by viruses. It binds to nearby cells and protects them from viral infection. **Complement** is a system of proteins that, during infection, enhances the immune response and inflammation. Complement also opsonizes pathogens – makes them more 'tasty' – so that they become easier targets for phagocytes.

• Fever

The abnormally high temperature that occurs with some infections serves to inhibit bacterial multiplication and speed up the rate of repair by body tissues.

Specific defences: the immune system

The immune system consists of macrophages and lymphocytes found particularly in the lymphatic system, but also in the cardiovascular system. It produces a highly targeted and specific defence system that is both adaptive and flexible. It is triggered by markers called **antigens** that are carried by pathogens and abnormal normal body cells. Immune system cells retain a memory of antigens, so that should the same pathogen be encountered again, the immune system launches a rapid and highly effective strike to destroy it. The immune system has two parts: the humoral (or antibody-mediated) immune response, controlled by **B-lymphocytes**, and the cell-mediated immune response, controlled by **T-lymphocytes**. Both types of lymphocytes are produced in bone marrow and B-lymphocytes mature there while T-lymphocytes mature in the thymus gland. As lymphocytes mature, or become immunocompetent, each becomes capable of responding to a specific antigen. The mature lymphocytes then disperse to lymph nodes, the spleen and other lymph tissue. When the immune system is confronted by a pathogen for the first time, it takes several days to respond to it – this is the primary response – during which symptoms of illness may appear. Should the same pathogen invade again later, the immune system responds immediately. This explains why people rarely suffer the same disease twice because they have become immune to it.

Humoral immune response: B lymphocytes

When a pathogen, such as a bacterium, enters the body it is engulfed by a macrophage, which 'presents' the pathogen's antigen to a matching B lymphocyte in the lymph system that is primed to recognize that specific antigen. The B lymphocytes divide rapidly to produce cells that spread to the blood and tissues and release chemicals called antibodies that bind to the pathogen and mark it for destruction by phagocytes. Division of B lymphocytes also produces memory B-cells that remember the pathogen and respond strongly should it ever return.

Cell-mediated immune response: T lymphocytes

This part of the immune system responds well to cells invaded by viruses and cancer cells – both have altered antigens. Macrophages engulfing these cells 'present' antigens to T-lymphocytes. Lymphocytes multiply rapidly, producing both killer T-lymphocytes that lock onto their target and kill it with chemicals and memory T-cells that retain a memory of the antigen for future reference.

▼ *At the centre of lymphocyte cells is a large nucleus with chromatin (yellow).*

▲ B-lymphocyte   ▼ T-lymphocyte

Although the body can survive without nutrition or water for a period of time, it has an absolute requirement for a continuous supply of oxygen. The reasons for this are twofold. First, oxygen is needed by each one of the body's trillions of cells in order to release the energy that is locked up in glucose and other fuel molecules. This energy is needed to power the many reactions going on inside cells that allow them to operate as living units. Second, oxygen cannot be stored by the body. Energy is released from glucose, with the involvement of oxygen, in the mitochondria of cells by cell respiration (see pp. 6–7), a process that releases carbon dioxide (and water) as a waste product.

The source of oxygen is the air around the body. By volume, oxygen makes up some 21% of the atmosphere at sea level. However, it is unfeasible to absorb oxygen through the skin's surface and supply it to all body cells. Instead the respiratory system takes air into the body, and facilitates the entry of oxygen into the bloodstream which carries it to all body cells. At the same time, the respiratory system removes carbon dioxide – which would poison the body if allowed to accumulate – and expels it from the body into the atmosphere.

The respiratory system consists of the lungs (see pp. 76–77) – through which oxygen enters and carbon dioxide leaves the bloodstream – and the airways – the nose, pharynx (throat), larynx, trachea and bronchi – that carry the air between the lungs and the atmosphere and are described below. Air is sucked into, and pushed out of, the lungs through the action of breathing.

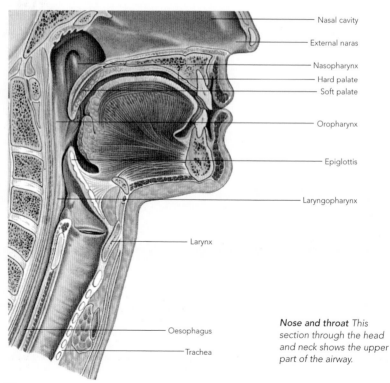

Nasal cavity

External naras

Nasopharynx

Hard palate

Soft palate

Oropharynx

Epiglottis

Laryngopharynx

Larynx

Oesophagus

Trachea

Nose and throat This section through the head and neck shows the upper part of the airway.

Nose

While air can be breathed in through either the mouth or nose, intake through the nose ensures that the air is filtered, moistened and warmed before it contacts the delicate tissues found inside the lungs. The nose consists of the external visible part, supported by cartilage, and the inner nasal cavity that is divided into left and right halves by the nasal septum. On the lateral side of each half there are three projecting 'ledges' formed by bones called the **conchae**, or turbinates. Like most of the airways, the nasal cavity is lined with ciliated mucous membrane that is well supplied with blood and secretes watery mucus. When air is breathed in through the external nares, or nostrils, the coarse hairs that guard the entrance to the nasal cavity remove larger dirt and dust particles. As the air passes over the conchae, it becomes turbulent and swirls over the nasal cavity lining. Heat from thin-walled blood vessels and moisture from the watery mucus warm and moisten the air. At the same time, dust and other particles become trapped in sticky mucus, which is wafted by the hair-like cilia to the throat, swallowed and digested by acidic gastric juice in the stomach which also kills any bacteria. Thus cleaned, air passes into the pharynx.

Pharynx

Looking like a short length of garden hose, the pharynx or throat, links the nose to the larynx. It provides a pathway not only for air, but also for food passing to the oesophagus. The pharynx has three continuous sections: the **nasopharynx** runs from the internal nares to the soft palate, the **oropharynx** connects with the back of the throat and the **laryngopharynx** divides into two parts – the anterior larynx and the posterior oesophagus.

Larynx

The funnel-shaped larynx, or voice box, is about 5 cm (2 in) long and links the pharynx to the trachea. Its structure and role in sound production are described on pp. 80–81. The **epiglottis** – the leaf-shaped flap of cartilage that is hinged at the superior, anterior edge of the larynx – folds posteriorly over the entrance to the larynx during swallowing (see pp. 84–85) to prevent food going 'the wrong way' towards the lungs.

Trachea

The trachea, or windpipe, is about 11 cm (4 in) long and runs behind the sternum to link the larynx to the lungs. It is reinforced by up to 20 C-shaped pieces of cartilage that prevent it from collapsing when air is sucked into the lungs. The open part of the 'C' occurs where the trachea adjoins the oesophagus, which runs parallel and posterior to the trachea. The tracheal epithelium secretes mucus which traps dust and cilia propel the dirt-laden mucus to the throat where it is swallowed. At its inferior end, the trachea branches into two bronchi which enter the lungs and branch repeatedly (see pp. 76–77).

▲ *Bronchial tree This false-colour bronchograph clearly shows the bronchial tree in a human lung. The airways in the lungs resemble an upside-down tree in which the trachea is the trunk, the bronchi are the main branches and the smaller bronchi and bronchioles form the branches and twigs.*

LUNGS AND GAS EXCHANGE

While the rest of the respiratory system is concerned with conveying air in and out of the body, the function of the lungs is to get oxygen into, and carbon dioxide out of, the bloodstream. Roughly cone shaped, the two lungs fill most of the thoracic cavity apart from the central mediastinum, which contains the heart, major blood vessels, trachea, bronchi and oesophagus. The apex of each lung extends above the clavicle, while its base rests on the diaphragm, the sheet of muscle that separates the thorax from the abdomen and plays a key role in breathing (see pp. 78–79). The lungs are surrounded and protected by the rib cage, formed by the sternum and ribs,

and the thoracic section of the vertebral column. Surrounding each lung is a double pleural membrane, or pleura: the **outer pleura** lines the inside of the thoracic cavity and the superior surface of the diaphragm and the **inner pleura** covers the lungs. Pleural fluid secreted by the pleural membranes ensures that during breathing the lungs slide painlessly over the thoracic wall. Each lung is divided into lobes by surface fissures: the right lung has two fissures and three lobes while the left lung has one fissure and two lobes and is smaller than its partner because of an indentation in its medial surface called the cardiac notch, which provides room for the heart.

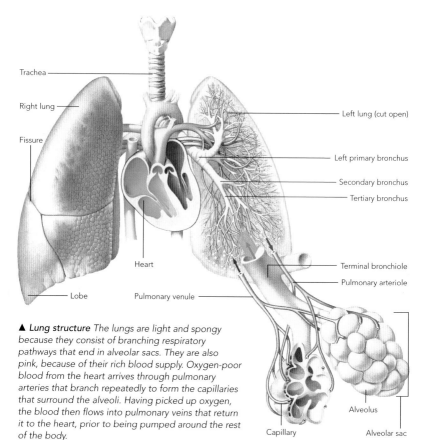

Trachea

Right lung

Fissure

Left lung (cut open)

Left primary bronchus

Secondary bronchus

Tertiary bronchus

Heart

Terminal bronchiole

Pulmonary arteriole

Lobe

Pulmonary venule

Capillary

Alveolus

Alveolar sac

▲ **Lung structure** The lungs are light and spongy because they consist of branching respiratory pathways that end in alveolar sacs. They are also pink, because of their rich blood supply. Oxygen-poor blood from the heart arrives through pulmonary arteries that branch repeatedly to form the capillaries that surround the alveoli. Having picked up oxygen, the blood then flows into pulmonary veins that return it to the heart, prior to being pumped around the rest of the body.

Bronchi and bronchioles

As already described on pp. 74–75, the trachea divides at its inferior end into two bronchi which each enter the lungs at an indentation called the **hilus**, which is also the entry and exit point for the pulmonary blood supply. Inside the lungs, each bronchus divides to form the secondary bronchi. These divide to form the tertiary bronchi, which in turn split into smaller bronchi and even smaller bronchioles no more than 1 mm (0.04 in) wide. These further subdivide into terminal bronchioles c.0.5 mm (0.02 in) wide, of which there are about 30,000 in each lung. Terminal bronchioles subdivide into two or more respiratory bronchioles that terminate in alveolar sacs, which resemble bunches of grapes. Each sac consists of a number of alveoli and it is through these that oxygen and carbon dioxide are exchanged.

Alveoli and gas exchange

The 300 million alveoli in both lungs provide a surface area for gas exchange of c.70 sq m (750 sq ft), or 35 times the surface area of the skin, crammed into a space no larger than a shopping bag. This large surface ensures that sufficient oxygen can be taken into the body to satisfy the demands of 100 trillion cells. Each alveolus is covered by a network of pulmonary blood capillaries. Its inner surface is covered by a thin film of fluid that contains a surfactant which prevents the alveoli from collapsing. The wall of the alveolus and that of the blood capillary adjacent to it forms the respiratory membrane. Oxygen diffuses across the membrane down a concentration gradient: with high oxygen levels in the alveolus and low oxygen in the blood it moves from the alveolus to the blood. Carbon dioxide moves in the opposite direction: with high carbon dioxide levels in the blood and low in the alveolus it moves from the former to the latter. The constant inflow of oxygen-rich air into the lungs, and the removal of oxygen-rich blood from the lungs, maintains these concentration gradients. The distance across the respiration membrane from the inside of the alveolus to the inside of the blood capillary is only 0.001 mm (0.00004 in), ensuring that diffusion can happen rapidly. Diffusion is aided by the fluid layer of the alveolus in which oxygen dissolves prior to crossing the respiratory membrane. Once in the blood, oxygen is carried by red blood cells (see pp. 64–65) to the tissues where oxygen passes into cells and waste carbon dioxide moves in the opposite direction.

Air rich in CO_2

Air rich in O_2

O_2 in blood

Capillary

Pulmonary arteriole

CO_2 in blood

Pulmonary venule

CO_2 dissolved in moist film

O_2 dissolved in moist film

▲ *Gas exchange in the alveolus* This diagram shows how carbon dioxide diffuses out of the blood and into the alveoli, while oxygen diffuses out of the alveoli and into the blood.

BREATHING

Air is constantly moved in and out of the lungs by a process called breathing (or ventilation). The normal breathing rate at rest is between 12 and 18 times a minute, but this rate increases during exercise to satisfy the increased oxygen needs of muscles. Apart from their bronchi, air sacs and blood vessels, lungs consist of elastic connective tissue and do not possess the muscles that could perform ventilation. Instead, their innate elasticity enables the lungs to follow the movement of the thoracic cavity in order to draw in or expel air. The lungs are effectively sealed inside the thorax by the thorax wall and diaphragm: the only opening is through the bronchi and trachea. The pleural fluid found between the paired pleural membranes lining the thorax and covering the lungs has an adhesive function, ensuring that as the thorax gets larger or smaller it pulls or pushes the elastic lungs so they too change in volume. The prime mover of breathing is the diaphragm, with the intercostal muscles between the ribs playing an assisting function. When the external intercostals contract, they raise the ribcage upwards and outwards. When their antagonists the internal intercostals contract, they pull the ribcage downwards and inwards.

Inhalation and exhalation
During inhalation (or inspiration), air is breathed in. The dome-shaped diaphragm contracts and pushes the underlying abdominal organs downwards while the external intercostal muscles contract and elevate the ribcage. As a result of these two actions, the volume inside the thorax increases and so – as described by Boyle's Law – the pressure inside the thorax decreases. Since the lungs follow the movements of the thorax, the volume of the lungs increases and their pressure decreases below that of the atmosphere outside the body. This negative pressure differential causes air to be sucked into the lungs. During quiet breathing, such as when someone is sitting at a desk, the diaphragm does most of the work, with the external intercostals only coming into play when that person becomes more active, and their rate and depth of breathing increase.

During exhalation, or expiration, air is breathed out. The diaphragm relaxes and is pushed upwards into a dome shape by the underlying abdominal organs. The ribs move downwards and inwards. Both actions cause the volume of the thoracic cavity to decrease and the naturally elastic lungs follow suit. The pressure inside the lungs increases above atmospheric pressure and air is forced out. During quiet breathing, once again, most of the work is done by the diaphragm. During forced exhalation, when a person is exercising vigorously, the internal intercostals come into play by actively returning the ribcage to its downwards position.

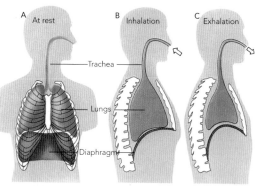

▲ *Inhalation and exhalation* The diaphragm contracts during inhalation and relaxes during exhalation.

Lung volumes
The lungs never completely empty: if they did, they would collapse and it would prove difficult to reinflate them. This means that the lungs are not completely flushed out and refilled with 'fresh' air with each breath. Instead, breathing refreshes air remaining in the lungs by adding more oxygen and removing carbon dioxide. The volume of air inhaled and exhaled with each breath depends on the

age and sex of the individual and their fitness. Doctors and other health specialists use certain respiratory volumes (*see* chart below) to assess their patients' health. Respiratory volumes are measured using a spirometer, an instrument that measures the volume of air passing in and out through a mouthpiece.

Control of breathing

The respiratory centre, in the medulla oblongata of the brain, automatically controls the breathing muscles through the phrenic nerve to the diaphragm and through the many intercostal nerves to the intercostal muscles. It can also make use of the accessory muscles of respiration when they are required.

The respiratory centre has two sources of information about breathing – the degree to which the lungs are stretched and the level of carbon dioxide in the bloodstream.

The stretching of the lungs through inspiration is detected by branches of the vagus nerve, which reflexly inhibit inspiration and allow expiration to take place. The fluctuations in the level of carbon dioxide are detected by nerve endings in the aorta and carotid arteries. An increase in carbon dioxide causes an increase in acidity of the blood and this stimulates the respiratory rate – a condition known as hyperpnea.

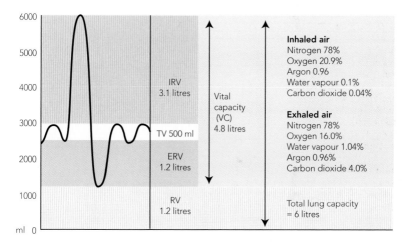

▲ *Lung volumes*
Respiratory volumes and respiratory capacities – combinations of particular respiratory volumes – are used to assess a person's respiratory health. The figures given here apply to a healthy male.
• Tidal volume (TV) is the volume of air that is inhaled and exhaled with each breath during quiet breathing.
• Inspiratory reserve volume (IRV) is the volume of air that can be forcibly inhaled in addition to TV.
• Expiratory reserve volume (ERV) is the volume of air that can be forcibly exhaled in addition to TV.
• Residual volume (RV) is the air that remains in the lungs after the most forceful exhalation.
• Inspiratory capacity (IC) is the sum of TV + IRV, and is the total amount of air that can be inhaled forcibly.
• Functional reserve capacity (FRC) is the sum of RV + ERV and is the amount of air remaining in the lungs after exhalation during quiet breathing.
• Vital capacity (VC) is the sum of TV + IRV + ERV and is the total volume of air that can be inhaled and exhaled.
• Total lung capacity is the sum of IRV + TV + ERV + RV. It is the total volume of air in fully inflated lungs.

In the figure:
- 6000, 5000, 4000, 3000, 2000, 1000, 0 ml
- IRV 3.1 litres
- TV 500 ml
- ERV 1.2 litres
- RV 1.2 litres
- Vital capacity (VC) 4.8 litres

Inhaled air
Nitrogen 78%
Oxygen 20.9%
Argon 0.96
Water vapour 0.1%
Carbon dioxide 0.04%

Exhaled air
Nitrogen 78%
Oxygen 16.0%
Water vapour 1.04%
Argon 0.96%
Carbon dioxide 4.0%

Total lung capacity = 6 litres

SPEECH AND BREATHING

The feature that distinguishes humans from other animals is the ability to communicate using speech sounds produced by the controlled release of exhaled breath though the vocal cords in the larynx and modified by tongue and lips. In addition, other respiratory movements produce sounds such as coughing and hiccuping.

Larynx and vocal cords

The larynx, or voice box, is situated superior to the trachea and can be felt as a firm projection in the anterior neck. It consists of nine pieces of cartilage and their associated muscles, held together by ligaments. These pieces of cartilage are the ring-shaped **cricoid cartilage** that attaches the larynx to the trachea; the **thyroid cartilage** and the paired **arytenoid cartilages** that anchor the vocal cords, the folds of fibrous tissue that stretch from the anterior to the posterior sides of the larynx; the **epiglottis**, the leaf-shaped cartilage flap that folds over the larynx and prevents food going 'the wrong way' towards the lungs during swallowing, and the paired **cuneiform** and **corniculate cartilages** that comprise part of the lateral and posterior walls of the larynx. In men, the anterior prominence of the thyroid cartilage can be felt in the neck as the so-called 'Adam's apple'.

There are two pairs of vocal cords. The upper pair, the **vestibular folds** or false vocal cords, do not play a part in sound production but help prevent food being inhaled. The lower pairs of true vocal cords are responsible for sound production. Between the true vocal cords is an opening called the **glottis**. This stays open during normal breathing.

Sound and speech production

Sounds are produced by the larynx during exhalation. Laryngeal muscles attached to the arytenoid cartilages contract to pull the vocal cords together. The forcing of exhaled air between the closed vocal cords forces them to vibrate, setting up sound waves in the air in the pharynx, nasal cavity and the mouth. The tauter the vocal cords are pulled by the laryngeal muscles, the faster the vibrations (and shorter the wavelength of the sound waves) and the higher pitched the sounds. The slacker the vocal cords are pulled and the wider the glottis, the lower pitched the sounds. Men naturally have lower-pitched voices than women because their vocal cords are thicker (this change occurs at puberty) and so vibrate more slowly. The volume of sound depends on the force with which air is sent between the vocal cords. During shouting, for example, air is sent through the glottis

► *Section though the larynx*
This vertical section through the larynx shows its main cartilage plates and the laryngeal muscles.

Epiglottis

Vocal cord

Glottis

Arytenoid cartilage
Thyroid cartilage
Cricoid cartilage

Laryngeal muscles

Trachea; C-shaped cartilages

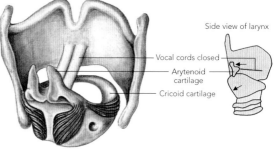

Side view of larynx

- Thyroid cartilage
- Vocal cords open
- Glottis open
- Arytenoid cartilage
- Laryngeal muscles

◀ *Sound production*
These two diagrams show how the movement of the arytenoid cartilages by the laryngeal muscles closes the glottis by pulling the vocal cords together and making them taut.

Posterior views of larynx

Side view of larynx

- Vocal cords closed
- Arytenoid cartilage
- Cricoid cartilage

with tremendous force and at high speed, producing sound waves of high amplitude with a resulting loud sound.

Raw sounds produced during breathing are then modified to produce the recognizable sounds in speech. The pharynx, nasal cavities and paranasal sinuses act as resonating chambers that amplify the sounds. Movements and shape-changes of the mouth cavity, tongue and lips produce recognizable vowels and consonants. Vowels are formed by altering the shape of the lips. Consonants are generated by a movement of the tip of the tongue to and from the back of the teeth or roof of the mouth, or by a rapid separation of the lips.

Speech requires the co-ordinated contraction of a number of different muscles including those that control breathing, the opening and closing of the vocal cords and the movement of the lips and tongue. Control of these muscles resides in Broca's (speech) area in the left cerebral hemisphere of the brain. Broca's area receives input from Wernicke's area about 'what is to be spoken'. Wernicke's area, in turn, receives input from other parts of the cerebrum including from the auditory cortex concerning spoken language and from the visual cortex about written language.

Other breathing movements

Several other processes, apart from

speech, may serve to modify the normal breathing pattern.

• **Coughing** is a reflex action that clears mucus and dust from the airways. A deep breath precedes the closing of the glottis. Muscles increase pressure in the thoracic cavity and air pressure builds up behind the vocal cords. These open suddenly, and air rushes up the bronchi, trachea and pharynx and out of the mouth, clearing the obstruction as it does so.

• **Sneezing** is similar to coughing except that the blast of air is directed out through the nasal cavity from which it removes irritating particles and mucus.

• **Hiccuping** is caused by an irritation of the diaphragm, perhaps by eating too quickly. The diaphragm contracts spasmodically, sucking air into the lungs in short bursts and making the vocal cords snap shut to produce the characteristic 'hiccup' sound.

• **Yawning** is probably stimulated by excess levels of carbon dioxide in the blood. It involves a deep inhalation with the mouth wide open, which 'flushes out' stale air from the lungs.

FOOD AND DIGESTION

Food – or, to be more specific, the nutrients contained in food – is essential for normal cell function and, therefore, to keep the body alive. Humans are driven to eat by appetite and hunger, both of which are controlled by the hypothalamus in the brain. The various nutrients contained in the food we eat provide cells with energy needed to power metabolism (see p. 8) and the raw materials required for growth and repair. Most foods contain a mixture of nutrients, although these nutrients are often 'locked' inside large molecules that cannot be used by the body because they are too big to be absorbed into the bloodstream. For absorption to occur, food has first to be digested by the digestive system, which works like an assembly line in reverse, converting complex nutrients into simpler ones. The process has four stages.

• **Ingestion** is the process of taking food or drink into the body through the mouth.

• **Digestion** is breaking down of complex nutrient molecules – mainly carbohydrates, fats, and proteins – into simpler ones.

• **Absorption** is the movement of the products of digestion, such as glucose or amino acids, from the alimentary canal into the bloodstream.

• **Egestion** is the elimination of indigestible material, such as fibre, as well as dead cells and bacteria from the body in the form of faeces.

Digestive system
The digestive system consists of two linked parts: the alimentary canal and the accessory digestive organs. The **alimentary canal** is essentially a tube, some 9 m (30 ft) long, that extends from the mouth to the anus, with its longest section – the intestines – packed into the abdominal cavity. The lining of the alimentary canal is continuous with the skin, so technically its cavity lies outside the body. The alimentary 'tube' consists of linked organs that each play their own part in digestion: mouth, pharynx, oesophagus, stomach, small intestine and large intestine. The **accessory digestive organs** consist of the teeth and tongue in the mouth and the salivary glands, liver, gall bladder and pancreas, which are all linked by ducts to the alimentary canal. The structure and function of the alimentary canal and its accessory organs are described in greater detail on pp. 84–93.

Digestion
As already explained, digestion is the breaking down of complex nutrients, such as fats, starches and proteins, into simple substances that can be absorbed by the body. The two forms of digestion – mechanical and chemical – work alongside each other. **Mechanical digestion** includes the cutting and grinding action of teeth and the churning action of the stomach's muscular walls. These actions physically break food up into smaller pieces, so that when food arrives in the small intestine – the main site of chemical digestion – it is in the form of a soup-like liquid called **chyme**. **Chemical digestion** involves the action of **enzymes** (see also pp. 8–9). These are biological catalysts that speed up reactions both inside and outside cells. Digestive enzymes are extracellular, working in the lumen of the alimentary canal. They accelerate by thousands or millions of times the breakdown of complex nutrients. Most enzymic activity takes place in the small intestine, although it also occurs in the mouth and the stomach.

Nutrients
Most food contains a mixture of carbohydrates, fats, proteins, vitamins, minerals and water. Vitamins and minerals – known as micronutrients because they are needed in small amounts – are typically absorbed unchanged in the small intestine, as is water. The other nutrients – macronutrients – usually need to be digested, unless they are ingested in simple form. Plant foods also contain fibre, consisting of cellulose and other indigestible elements of the plant's skeletal structure. Fibre is an essential element of the human diet because it adds bulk to food and gives gut wall muscles something to act against, speeding the movement of waste along the large intestine.

• **Carbohydrates**
Carbohydrates are important sources of energy. They divide into two groups:

polysaccharides (complex carbohydrates) that do not taste sweet and **sugars** (monosaccharides and disaccharides) that do. Complex carbohydrates, such as starch, are made up of long chains of glucose molecules. Initially, during digestion, starch is broken down into a disaccharide (two-sugar unit) called maltose, which is then broken down into individual glucose (monosaccharide) molecules. Other di-saccharides, such as sucrose (cane sugar) and lactose (milk sugar), taken in with food are broken down into their constituent simple sugars, glucose and fructose and glucose and galactose, respectively. These simple sugars are then absorbed.

• Proteins

Proteins perform a wide range of meta-bolic roles inside cells and are built up from building blocks called amino acids, which are absorbed following digestion. The proteins in food consist of long chains of amino acids, of which there are 20 types. Initially proteins are 'cut' into shorter lengths called peptides, a process that begins in the stomach. Then, in the small intestine, peptidases snip individual amino acids off the end of the peptide chains. The amino acids are then absorbed.

• Fats and oils

Also called lipids, fats and oils are required to help build cell membranes, insulate the body and provide an energy store. Fats and oils consist of molecules called **triglyc-erides**, each of which is made up of glycerol and three fatty acids. **Lipases** break down each tri-glyceride into two fatty acids and monoglycerides (glycerol attached to one fatty acid). These are then absorbed.

Lower end of oesophagus

Stomach

Liver

Pancreas

Hepatic portal vein

Large intestine

Small intestine

Appendix

Rectum

Anus

◀ *Digestive system This diagram shows the main parts of the digestive system. The mouth, pharynx and most of the oesophagus are not shown (see pp. 84–85).*

CHEWING AND SWALLOWING

Mouth and chewing

The mouth provides the entrance to both digestive systems. It is bounded by the lips, hard and soft palates, cheeks and tongue. Posteriorly, the mouth opens into the pharynx. The **lips** are flexible, muscular and highly sensitive flaps that guard the entrance to the mouth. The muscular **cheeks** extend from below the eye to the margin of the jaw. The hard **palate** forms the roof of the mouth, and is supported by bone; the soft **palate** is supported by muscle. The **tongue** is a muscular flap that occupies most of the mouth cavity when it is closed. Intrinsic muscles within the tongue change its shape, while extrinsic muscles, anchored to bone, protrude and retract the tongue. The tongue moves and mixes food during chewing and houses taste buds (*see* pp. 48–49) that detect tastes. The **teeth** provide a 'tool kit' of four types of teeth for grasping and breaking up food: chisel-shaped **incisors** grip food and cut it up into manageable pieces, pointed **canines** grip and pierce food, broad-crowned **premolar** teeth crush and chew it and large, broad-crowned teeth, the **molars**, at the back of the jaw, crush food with great force.

Food is ingested by the pulling action of the lips and the gripping and tearing of the incisors and canines. Once food is inside the mouth, the lips close and the cheeks flatten as the buccinator muscles contract. The masseter and temporalis (jaw) muscles open and close the jaws, enabling the premolar and molar teeth to crush and grind the food. At the same time, the sight, smell and presence of food in the mouth causes the reflex release into the mouth cavity of saliva from the salivary glands. Watery saliva contains **amylase**, an enzyme that breaks starch down to the disaccharide sugar maltose; mucus, to help to bind food particles together and lubricate their passage during swallowing, and **lysozyme**, an antibacterial substance. As the teeth crush food, the tongue mixes it, then pushes it against the hard palate to form a slippery package called a bolus and then pushes it backward toward the throat.

Swallowing

Swallowing has three stages.
• **The oral stage**, already described, occurs when the tongue pushes the food bolus towards the throat. It is under voluntary control, while the rest of the process is automatic, controlled by the autonomic nervous system and a swallowing centre in the brain.

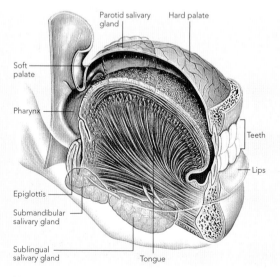

Parotid salivary gland
Hard palate
Soft palate
Pharynx
Teeth
Lips
Epiglottis
Submandibular salivary gland
Sublingual salivary gland
Tongue

The mouth This diagram shows the main features of the mouth – the tongue, cheeks and hard and soft palates – and the epiglottis and pharynx. Three pairs of salivary glands empty about 1.5 l (2.5 pt) of saliva through ducts into the mouth daily. These are the parotid glands in front of the ear, the sublingual glands just below the tongue and the submandibular glands just inside the mandible.

• **The pharyngeal stage** is triggered when the bolus touches the back of the throat. A wave of muscular contractions pushes the bolus into the oesophagus, breathing ceases temporarily and the epiglottis folds over the entrance to the larynx to stop food going towards the lungs.

• **The oesophageal stage** pushes food down the oesophagus by a wave of muscle contraction called peristalsis. Like much of the rest of the digestive system, the wall of the oesophagus contains both circular (inner) and longitudinal (outer) smooth muscle fibres. Circular muscle behind the bolus contracts, while that in front of the bolus relaxes, so food is pushed downwards as the waves of contraction and relaxation pass down the oesophagus. In addition, longitudinal muscles in front of the bolus contract, making the oesophagus wider and shorter. The journey time from pharynx to stomach is between 4 and 8 seconds.

Circular muscles contracted
Food bolus
Circular muscles relaxed
Longitudinal muscles contracted

◀ ▲ *Peristalsis These longitudinal sections through the oesophagus outline how the automatic, rhythmic muscular contraction of peristalsis pushes food from the throat to the stomach, as well as moving food in other parts of the digestive system.*

Oesophagus

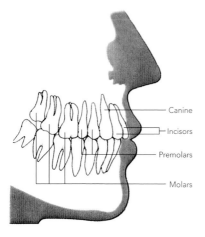

Canine
Incisors
Premolars
Molars

▲ *Permanent teeth Humans have two sets of teeth in their lifetime. The first set of 24 milk, or deciduous, teeth first appears at the age of six months and persists until late childhood. They are gradually pushed out and replaced by the larger set of 32 adult, or permanent, teeth that develop as the jaws get longer. In each half of each jaw there are two incisors, one canine, two premolars and three molars.*

Enamel
Blood capillary
Nerve
Pulp
Gum
Crown
Dentine
Cementum
Root
Periodontal ligament

▲ *Structure of a tooth The teeth are anchored in sockets in the upper and lower jaws and surrounded by the gums. The upper exposed part of the tooth is its crown and the lower part is its root. As this section shows, the crown is covered by enamel, the hardest material in the body. Beneath this is bone-like dentine which shapes the tooth and extends downwards into the roots. The inner, soft pulp cavity contains blood vessels and nerves: it produces dentine and provides sensations during chewing. The roots are held in place by cementum and the periodontal ligament within the tooth socket.*

STOMACH

The second stage of digestion takes place in the stomach. This J-shaped organ lies between, and connects, the lower end of the oesophagus and the duodenum, the first section of the small intestine. The stomach forms the widest, most elastic and most muscular part of the alimentary canal. This reflects its two main functions. First, it crushes food and churns it up with powerful gastric juices secreted by glands in its lining. Second, it provides a holding area that stores food for three to four hours and then releases it at a slow and steady rate as the small intestine becomes ready to process it. Without this storage area, food would be unable to move along the small intestine to be digested and absorbed efficiently.

Stomach structure

On average, an adult stomach is about 25 cm (10 in) long, but, thanks to its elasticity, its volume can vary greatly. When completely empty, the stomach is no bigger than a fist, with a volume of about 50 ml (1.7 fl oz) and its inner lining is thrown into deep folds called rugae. When completely full, after a large meal, its volume can increase to up to 4 l (7 pt) and the rugae disappear as the elastic stomach walls stretch.

The stomach has four regions: the **cardiac region** surrounds the opening of the oesophagus; the **fundus** is the upper, dome-shaped section; the **body** is the middle region and the **pylorus** is the funnel-shaped final section, linked to the duodenum by a ring of muscle called the pyloric sphincter.

The mucous membrane lining the inside of the stomach contains millions of deep gastric pits that contain gastric glands. These glands produce the components of gastric juice: **hydrochloric acid**, necessary to produce the harsh acid conditions inside the stomach; **pepsinogen**, which is turned into the active protein-digesting enzyme by hydrochloric acid; **intrinsic factor**, which is necessary for the absorption of the essential vitamin B_{12} by the small intestine, and, in children, the enzyme **rennin** which converts soluble milk protein into a curd that can be more easily digested. In addition, the glands also produce the hormone **gastrin** which is involved in co-ordinating digestion.

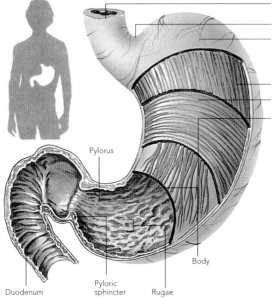

Oesophagus

Cardiac region

Fundus

Outer longitudinal muscle

Middle circular muscle

Inner oblique muscle

Pylorus

Duodenum

Pyloric sphincter

Rugae

Body

◀ *Stomach structure This section though the stomach shows the three muscle layers found in its wall; the rugae, or folds, that form when the stomach is empty; the stomach wall, which contains millions of gastric glands, and the pyloric sphincter which controls the release of food from the stomach following digestion.*

Gastric glands also secrete bicarbonate-rich (alkaline) mucus which covers the stomach's lining and protects it from self-digesting by pepsin and attack by hydrochloric acid. Lining cells are replaced every few days as they become worn by exposure to gastric juice.

In addition to layers of longitudinal and circular muscle, the stomach wall also contains an additional inner layer of oblique muscle. These muscle layers contract in turn to churn up food.

Digestion in the stomach

Some 2 l (3.5 pt) of gastric juice is secreted each day inside the stomach. Its hydrochloric acid produces an acidic environment of between pH 1.5 and 3.5, ideal for the action of pepsin (most enzymes work best at a neutral or slightly acid pH) which breaks down proteins to shorter chains of amino acids called polypeptides. Hydrochloric acid also destroys most bacteria that enter the stomach in food or drink. The release of gastric juice is co-ordinated to ensure that it is at its peak when food is about to, or has, entered the stomach. There are three overlapping phases of gastric secretion, as outlined below.

• **Cephalic phase** is the release of gastric juice under the control of the autonomic nervous system (ANS) triggered when the brain perceives the thought, sight, smell or taste of food.

• **Gastric phase** occurs when food arrives in the stomach. The stretching of the stomach wall causes the release of the hormone gastrin which targets the gastric glands that produce it and causes them to release more gastric juice.

• **Intestinal phase** is triggered by arrival of food in the duodenum. This inhibits the release of gastric juice so that the small intestine has time to process the current batch of food before the next one arrives from the stomach.

As food is pushed through the stomach by peristalsis, the waves of contraction become stronger and stronger until they reach the pylorus where they are powerful enough to crush and churn the food. As the ANS stimulates the release of gastric juice, so it increases gastric motility – the speed and strength of contractions of the stomach wall. The crushing of food and its mixing with gastric juice eventually produces a soup-like liquid called chyme. This is pushed against the closed pyloric sphincter, which opens slightly to allow squirts of chyme into the duodenum. Any larger, as yet untreated pieces of food are unable to pass through the small opening, and are recycled for further digestion. The stomach generally empties between two and four hours after a meal, longer if the meal has been very fatty.

Filling

Muscular contractions mix food with gastric juice as it enters the stomach.

Digestion

Strong contractions churn food as gastric juice digests it into chyme.

Emptying

The pyloric sphincter relaxes to allow liquid chyme into the duodenum.

▲ *Gastric filling and emptying This diagram shows the three phases of digestion in the stomach.*

SMALL INTESTINE AND PANCREAS

The intestines make up about 80% of the length of the alimentary canal. They have two sections and are coiled and folded to fit into the limited space inside the abdominal cavity. The small intestine carries out the major part of food digestion, as well as the absorption of the simple molecules that are the products of digestion. The large intestine plays no part in digestion but serves to absorb water and salts and convey undigested waste out of the body. Both are lined with slippery mucous membrane that secretes lubricating and protective mucus and both have layers of longitudinal and circular muscle in their walls that facilitate the movement of food or waste along their length by peristaltic and other movements. The structure of the small intestine, as well as that of the pancreas and gall bladder, both accessory digestive

organs, is described here. The digestion and absorption of food by the small intestine, and the structure and functions of the large intestine, are described on pp. 90–91.

Small intestine

The small intestine is the longest and most important part of the alimentary canal. It is between 6 and 7 m (20–23 ft) long in its relaxed state and about 2.5 cm (1 in) in diameter. It extends from the pyloric sphincter, which guards the exit from the stomach, to the ileocaecal sphincter, which guards the entrance to the large intestine. It has three parts: the duodenum, jejunum and ileum. The **duodenum** is 25 cm (10 in) long and receives partially digested food, called chyme, from the stomach; bile, a product of the liver, from the gall bladder

Jejunum

Common bile duct

Pancreatic duct

Ampulla of Vater

Villi

Longitudinal muscle layer

Circular muscle layer

Circular fold

Intestinal gland

Ileum

Branch of mesenteric artery

Branch of hepatic portal vein carries absorbed food to the liver

Duodenum

◀ *Duodenum and small intestine This section through the duodenum shows the structure of the small intestine, the opening through the ampulla of Vater of the common bile duct from the liver and the pancreatic duct from the pancreas. On the left are the jejunum and ileum, the other sections of the small intestine.*

▼ *Pancreas* *This section through the pancreas shows both exocrine and endocrine regions.*

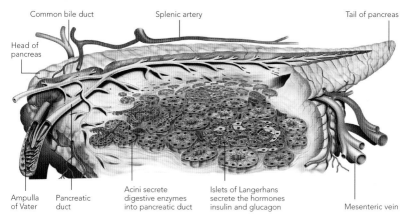

Common bile duct   Splenic artery   Tail of pancreas

Head of pancreas

Ampulla of Vater

Pancreatic duct

Acini secrete digestive enzymes into pancreatic duct

Islets of Langerhans secrete the hormones insulin and glucagon

Mesenteric vein

along the common bile duct and enzyme-containing pancreatic juice from the pancreas. The common bile duct and pancreatic duct merge just before entering the small intestine, so their secretions flow through a common opening. The **jejunum** is about 2.5 m (8 ft) long and links the duodenum to the **ileum**, which is about 3.6 m (12 ft) long and is where most absorption of nutrients takes place.

The effectiveness of the small intestine in both digestion and absorption is increased by three structural features: circular folds, villi and microvilli. **Circular folds** (or plicae circularis) extend around the circumference of the small intestine, increasing its surface area and slowing the flow of chyme, so giving more time for digestion. **Villi** are tiny finger-like processes about 1 mm (0.04 in) long. They significantly increase the surface area through which food can be absorbed. **Microvilli** are microscopic folds that cover the outer surface of intestinal cells – including those covering the villi – and carry digestive enzymes – called brush border enzymes – that complete the final stages of digestion. These three features give the small intestine a surface area of more than 200 sq m (2,150 sq ft), equivalent to the floor area of an average two-storey house.

Pancreas

This long organ lies almost horizontally below the stomach. Exocrine cells, arranged in clusters called acini, secrete pancreatic juice which passes along the pancreatic duct and empties into the duodenum through the ampulla of Vater. The 1.5 l (2.5 pt) of pancreatic juice produced daily contains a number of enzymes. It is alkaline and helps to neutralize the acidic chyme arriving from the stomach, thereby helping to provide an optimal pH for the action of pancreatic and intestinal enzymes. The endocrine portions of the pancreas, the **Islets of Langerhans**, secrete insulin and glucagon, two hormones that control glucose levels in blood (*see* pp. 56–57).

Gall bladder

About 10 cm (4 in) in length, this muscular sac is located on the posterior surface of the liver. It stores and concentrates bile, a greenish-yellow liquid, of which about 1 l (1.75 pt) is produced by the liver daily. Bile contains water, cholesterol, bile pigments (the waste product of the breakdown of haemoglobin from red blood cells) and bile salts that play a part in fat digestion. Bile is carried from the liver to the gall bladder by the common hepatic duct.

INTESTINES

Digestion in the small intestine

The digestion of food in the small intestine utilizes enzymes from two sources – pancreatic juice secreted by the pancreas and the brush border enzymes attached to the microvilli that project from the epithelial cells lining the small intestine. Bile from the gall bladder does not contain enzymes but still has a key role in digestion.

When chyme arrives in the duodenum from the stomach, it triggers the release of two hormones – cholecystokinin (CCK) and secretin – by the intestinal wall. These hormones stimulate pancreatic juice secretion. Pancreatic juice travels along the pancreatic duct and empties into the duodenum through the ampulla of Vater. It contains a number of enzymes, although its protein-digesting proteases are not activated until they reach the small intestine. This prevents the self-digestion of the pancreas. CCK also stimulates release of bile from the gall bladder and this is squirted into the duodenum at the same time as pancreatic juice and through the same opening. The bile salts in bile emulsify fat globules in food, breaking them up into tiny droplets. These droplets present a very large surface area for pancreatic lipase, the enzyme that digests fats, to act on. Pancreatic juice is alkaline, as is the watery intestinal juice that is secreted by glands in the small intestine wall. This helps to neutralize acidic chyme and provide an optimal, slightly alkaline pH for the activity of both pancreatic and brush border enzymes. The action of these enzymes is shown in the table opposite.

Absorption by the small intestine

Digestion by brush border enzymes yields molecules that are small enough to be absorbed by villi, the finger-like projections that cover the small intestine, especially those in the ileum. Glucose and other simple sugars, amino acids and nucleic acid breakdown products are carried through the cells covering the villi, pass into the blood capillaries inside them and are carried by the hepatic portal vein to the liver for processing (see pp. 92–93). Fatty acids and monoglycerides (a combination of one fatty acid molecule

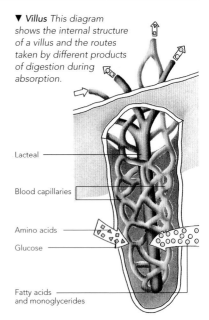

▼ *Villus This diagram shows the internal structure of a villus and the routes taken by different products of digestion during absorption.*

Lacteal

Blood capillaries

Amino acids

Glucose

Fatty acids and monoglycerides

and a glycerol molecule) pass into the epithelial cells of villi, where they are converted back into triglycerides (oils), and then into the lacteals, tiny branches of the lymphatic system (see pp. 70–71). The lymphatic system carries triglycerides away from the ileum and deposits them in the bloodstream. Minerals and vitamins are also absorbed, as is about 95% of the 9 l (16 pt) of water that enters the small intestine each day.

Food spends between 3 to 6 hours in the small intestine. Localized contractions of circular muscles in the intestinal wall move chyme backwards and forwards – a process called segmentation – which optimizes both digestion and absorption. The rhythmic contraction of peristalsis is also seen, especially when digestion and absorption are completed and undigested matter is pushed towards the large intestine.

Large intestine

The large intestine is about 1.5 m (5 ft) long and 6.5 cm (2.5 in) in diameter: it extends from the ileocaecal valve to the anus. It is divided up into four parts: the caecum, colon, rectum and anal canal. The pouch-like caecum lies just inferior to the ileocaecal valve that maintains a one-way flow from the small intestine to the large . The colon – the main part of the large intestine – has four regions: the ascending colon passes up the right-hand side of the abdominal cavity, the transverse colon passes across the abdominal cavity just inferior to the liver, the descending colon passes down the right-hand side of the abdominal cavity and the S-shaped sigmoid colon joins the rectum. The longitudinal muscle of the colon is reduced to three strips, called taeniae, that pull the colon into pockets called haustra. The rectum is about 20 cm (8 in) long and leads to the 3 cm (1.2 in) long anal canal which opens to the outside through the anus.

The large intestine does not have a digestive role. It processes the material arriving from the small intestine – undigested food, bile pigments and dead cells – and turns it into semi-solid faeces that are eliminated from the body. It does this by absorbing water and salts. The large intestine also contains billions of bacteria that feed on undigested material and release some B and K vitamins that are absorbed across the intestinal wall.

Some 1.5 l (2.5 pt) of waste arrives each day in the colon from the small intestine. Most of the time, muscles in the intestinal wall contract sluggishly to push waste material slowly along the colon so that water and salts can be absorbed and the waste converted into faeces. About three times a day, after meals, a more powerful peristaltic wave – triggered by the arrival of food in the stomach – pushes faeces into the sigmoid colon where they are stored until defecation occurs. Every 500 ml (1 pt) of waste entering the colon produces about 150 g (5 oz) of faeces. The journey from ileocaecal valve to sigmoid colon takes between 12 and 36 hours, depending on the type of food.

The arrival of faeces in the rectum stretches its wall. This triggers a reflex action, controlled by the autonomic nervous system, that pushes the faeces into the anal canal and relaxes the internal and external sphincters that guard the anal opening. At the same time a person has a conscious awareness of the need to defecate. The muscles of the rectum then contract to push the faeces out. However, the defecation reflex can be overridden by conscious intervention and the external sphincter is closed.

▼ *Action of pancreatic and intestinal enzymes in the small intestine. Nutrients in* **bold italics** *are those that are absorbed by the small intestine.*

Secretion	Enzyme	Action
Bile from the liver	—	Bile salts emulsify fats into small droplets
Pancreatic juice	Amylase	Breaks down starch into maltose
	Trypsin	Breaks down proteins into peptides
		Converts inactive chymotrypsinogen into active enzyme chymotrypsin
	Chymotrypsin	Breaks down proteins into peptides
	Lipase	Breaks down fats and oils droplets into *fatty acids* and *monoglycerides*
	Carboxypeptidase	Breaks down peptides into *amino acids*
	Nucleases	Break down DNA and RNA into nucleotides
Brush border enzymes on intestinal epithelial cells	Enterokinase	Converts inactive trypsinogen into active enzyme trypsin
	Peptidases	Break down peptides into *amino acids*
	Nucleosidases	Break down nucleotides into *nitrogenous bases, pentoses* and *phosphates*
	Maltase	Breaks down maltose into *glucose*
	Sucrase	Breaks down sucrose into *glucose* and *fructose*
	Lactase	Breaks down lactose into *glucose* and *galactose*

LIVER AND METABOLISM

Weighing 1.5 kg (3.3 lb), the liver is the body's largest internal organ. The wedge-shaped liver occupies much of the top right-hand side of the abdominal cavity, immediately under the diaphragm. Its deep red colour is indicative of the large volume of blood that passes through it. The liver's 500 metabolic and regulatory functions play a key part in homeostasis by ensuring that the blood's composition remains constant. While the liver's only direct role in digestion is to produce bile, many of its functions involve processing the products of digestion after they arrive from the small intestine.

Liver structure

The basic units of the liver are the billions of **hepatocytes**, or liver cells, that process nutrients, produce bile, destroy poisons and secrete substances. They are arranged not at random but into highly organized, microscopic structures called lobules. Each **lobule** consists of vertical plates of hepatocytes that radiate from a central core (*see below*). At each of the six corners of a lobule there are three vessels: a branch of the hepatic portal vein that delivers nutrient-rich blood, a branch of

the hepatic artery that delivers oxygen-rich blood and a branch of the bile duct. Blood from both blood vessels mixes inside blood spaces called **sinusoids** that run between the plates of hepatocytes. It then empties into the central vein that runs along the core of the lobule before emptying into a hepatic vein. As blood flows along the sinusoid, hepatocytes remove oxygen, as well as nutrients and other substance to be processed, and add secretory products, nutrients released from store and waste products. Sinusoids contain macrophages, called **Kupffer cells**, that engulf worn-out red blood cells, debris and bacteria. Bile produced by the hepatocytes flows along the bile **canaliculi** that run between plates of hepatocytes and collects in a branch of the bile duct. It is then carried by the bile duct to be stored in the gall bladder.

Major functions of the liver

By carrying out their 500 or so metabolic functions, the hepatocytes control the chemical composition of the blood. The main functions are described below.

• Blood glucose regulation

Cells need a constant supply of glucose to provide energy to drive their metabolic reactions so it is essential that glucose levels stay relatively constant. If blood glucose levels are high, after a meal, the liver sequesters glucose and stores it in the form of the polysaccharide glycogen. If levels are too low, between meals, the liver converts glycogen to glucose, which is released

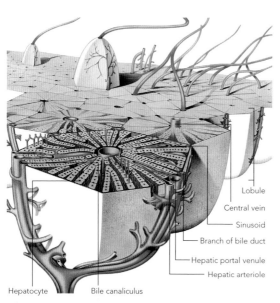

Lobule
Central vein
Sinusoid
Branch of bile duct
Hepatic portal venule
Hepatic arteriole
Hepatocyte   Bile canaliculus

◀ *Liver lobules This magnified view inside the liver shows the hexagonal lobules that make up its structure. Each consists of radiating sheets of hepatocytes between which run the blood-carrying sinusoids and bile-carrying canaliculi.*

into the blood. This regulatory process also involves the mediation of the pancreatic hormones insulin and glucagon (see pp. 56–57).

• Fat metabolism
If liver glycogen stores are full, the liver converts excess glucose to fat, which can be stored either in the liver or in adipose tissue. The liver also produces cholesterol, a precursor of some steroid hormones and a component of the outer plasma membrane of cells.

• Mineral storage
Iron and copper, both needed to make the haemoglobin inside red blood cells, are stored inside hepatocytes.

• Vitamin storage
Vitamins A, D and B_{12} are amongst the vitamins stored by the liver. The liver can hold up to four months' supply of vitamins D and B_{12}, and about two years' supply of vitamin A.

• Protein metabolism
Excess amino acids, the building blocks of proteins, cannot be stored in the body. The liver processes the excess by deaminating the amino acids to form urea, a nitrogen-containing waste which is carried to the kidneys to be excreted

in urine. In addition, the liver produces plasma proteins and fibrinogen found in blood (see pp. 64–65).

• Bile production
Bile consists of bile pigments derived from the breakdown of red blood cells, bile salts derived from cholesterol, cholesterol itself and fats. Bile salts play a part in fat digestion in the small intestine and are then absorbed back into the bloodstream, returned to the liver and reused. The other bile components are excreted with the faeces.

• Hormone breakdown
The liver removes hormones from the blood and breaks them down.

• Detoxification
Poisonous substances, such as alcohol, that have been inhaled or ingested are detoxified by the liver, which converts them into harmless substances that can be excreted by the kidneys.

• Heat generation
The many metabolic reactions going on inside the hepatocytes generate a considerable amount of heat. This is distributed around the body by the blood and helps to maintain a constant body temperature.

▶ *Liver's blood supply*
The liver has two blood supplies: 20% is provided by the hepatic artery which supplies oxygen-rich blood; 80% arrives along the hepatic portal vein that delivers blood that is poor in oxygen but rich in nutrients and other materials from the small intestine. A portal system is one that carries blood from one organ to another rather than returning it to the heart. The hepatic artery and hepatic portal vein enter the liver midway down its posterior surface. Inside the liver, the oxygen-rich and oxygen-poor/nutrient-rich blood is mixed. 'Processed' blood

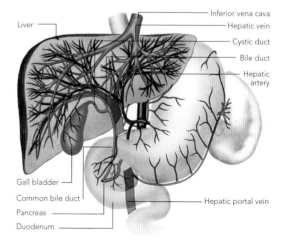

Liver — Inferior vena cava — Hepatic vein — Cystic duct — Bile duct — Hepatic artery — Gall bladder — Common bile duct — Pancreas — Duodenum — Hepatic portal vein

leaves the liver through the hepatic veins that immediately empty into

the inferior vena cava which returns the blood to the heart.

KIDNEYS

The two kidneys play a vital role in homeostasis by processing the blood to produce a waste fluid called urine which is expelled from the body. By so doing, the kidneys are carrying out two major functions. The first is excretion of unwanted, and potentially poisonous, metabolic wastes produced by cells, notably urea, a nitrogenous waste product generated by the deamination of amino acids in the liver. The second is osmoregulation, the removal of excess water and salts (such as sodium and potassium salts) in order to maintain constant levels of water and salts in the blood and other body fluids.

Kidney structure

The two bean-shaped kidneys lie high in the posterior abdominal cavity, partially protected by the lowest ribs. An adult kidney is about 12 cm (5 in) long and 6 cm (2.4 in) wide, and is protected by a thin outer capsule. On the medial side of each kidney is an indentation (or hilus) through which nerves and a renal artery enter the kidney and a renal vein and urethra leave it. A section though the kidney reveals that it consists of three zones: an outer renal cortex, a middle renal medulla and a central renal pelvis. A flattened, funnel-shaped tube collects urine and directs it into the ureter.

Nephrons and urine production

Running between the cortex and medulla of each kidney are about 1 million microscopic nephrons. These are the 'filtering units' of the kidney that produce urine. Each nephron consists of a glomerulus and a renal tubule, comprising a Bowman's capsule, proximal and

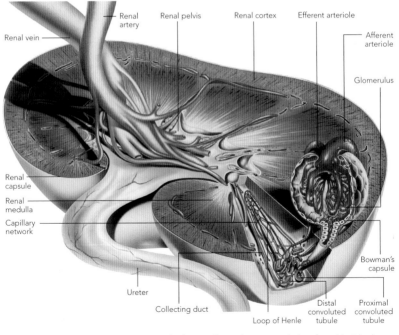

Renal vein — Renal artery — Renal pelvis — Renal cortex — Efferent arteriole — Afferent arteriole — Glomerulus — Renal capsule — Renal medulla — Capillary network — Ureter — Collecting duct — Loop of Henle — Distal convoluted tubule — Proximal convoluted tubule — Bowman's capsule

▲ *Kidney structure*
This diagram shows a longitudinal section through a kidney, with a detailed,

magnified view of one the microscopic nephrons – each consisting of a glomerulus and a renal

tubule – found inside the cortex and medulla of each kidney.

distal convoluted tubules, a loop of Henle and a collecting duct (see diagram, below left). The glomerulus is a cluster of 'leaky' blood capillaries. Blood enters the glomerulus through an afferent arteriole and leaves through a narrower, efferent arteriole. The difference in diameters produces high blood pressure inside the glomerulus, which forces fluid (but not cells or plasma proteins) from the blood into the cup-shaped Bowman's capsule. This fluid contains not just wastes, but also glucose, amino acids, water and other material that the body needs to retain. As this filtrate passes along the proximal convoluted (twisted) tubule, glucose, amino acids and most salt and water are reabsorbed into the blood flowing through the surrounding capillary network. Further concentration and reabsorption continues in the loop of Henle and the distal convoluted tubule to produce a fluid, now called urine, that arrives in a collecting duct that receives input from several nephrons. The permeability of the collecting duct wall to water is mediated by the pituitary gland hormone ADH. In this way, urine can be further concentrated should the body need to retain more water or left dilute if the body's water content is near to normal. Urine then passes into the renal pelvis and onwards to the bladder for expulsion (see pp. 96–97). About 95% of urine consists of water: the remaining 5% consists mainly of nitrogenous wastes, salts and metabolized hormones. Its yellow colour is produced by urochrome, a breakdown product of haemoglobin.

The importance of the kidneys in homeostasis is highlighted by the amount of blood they process daily. The renal arteries deliver about 25% of the cardiac output to the kidneys regardless of how active the body is: this amounts to about 1.2 l (2 pt) per minute, or 1,800 l (3,150 pt) per day. Each day 180 l (315 pt) of fluid is filtered from blood plasma through glomerular capillaries and into Bowman's capsules: only 1%, amounting to c.1.5 l (2.5 pt) leaves the body as urine. The body's entire blood supply is processed by the kidneys about 60 times every day.

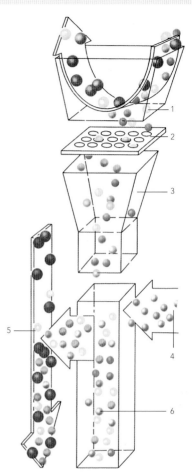

▲ **The filtering mechanism** Blood flows at high pressure (above) through the capillaries of the Bowman's capsule (**1**) and only small molecules are forced through the walls (**2**) into the first part of the nephron (**3**). The filtrate passes down the proximal tubule, which secretes further metabolites and salts (**4**) and reabsorbs water, sodium, essential salts, glucose and amino acids into the blood (**5**). The loop of Henle and distal tubule are concerned with both the reabsorption of water and the maintenance of the overall acid-alkaline balance of the body. Unwanted salts, urea and water are left as urine (**6**).

BLADDER AND URINATION

Ureters, bladder and urethra

Urine is produced by the two kidneys in a constant trickle of about 1 ml (0.05 fl oz) per minute. The other organs of the urinary system – the two ureters, the bladder and the urethra – serve to channel and store urine until a convenient time is found for its release and then transport urine to the outside of the body.

Each **ureter** is a hollow tube, between 25 and 30 cm (10–12 in) long, with a wall that contains both longitudinal and circular layers of smooth muscle. It begins as an extension of the renal pelvis and then travels vertically downwards to open in the posterior wall of the bladder, an arrangement that prevents backflow of urine. Urine is pushed along the ureters by rhythmic contraction of the smooth muscle layers called peristalsis (see pp. 84–85).

The **bladder** is a 'storage bag' that has a muscular, highly elastic wall. When empty, just after urination, it can be as small as a plum. As it fills, it can hold 300–400 ml (10–13 fl oz) of urine before a person feels a conscious desire to urinate,

and can hold double that volume before the person has an urgent need to urinate. The wall of the bladder contains layers of smooth muscle fibres that contract to squeeze out urine.

The thin-walled, muscular **urethra** leaves the base of the bladder to carry urine to the outside. In adult males, it is about 20 cm (8 in) long and opens at the tip of the penis. In adult females, it is about 4 cm (2 in) long and opens halfway between the clitoris and the vaginal opening. In the bladder wall at its junction with the urethra is a ring of smooth muscle, the internal urethral sphincter, that is under involuntary control. Where the urethra passes through the pelvic floor muscles there is an external urethral sphincter that is made of skeletal muscle.

Bladder filling and emptying

As the bladder fills with urine, its inner folds, or rugae, start to disappear. As this happens, stretch receptors in the muscular wall detect increasing tension in the wall and sends nerve impulses to the spinal cord. When the bladder contains 200–300

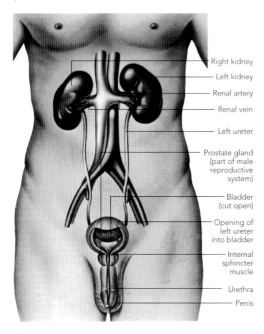

Right kidney

Left kidney

Renal artery

Renal vein

Left ureter

Prostate gland (part of male reproductive system)

Bladder (cut open)

Opening of left ureter into bladder

Internal sphincter muscle

Urethra

Penis

◀ *Urinary system This diagram shows the organs that make up the male urinary system, a system that is located in the abdominal cavity. The two kidneys (kidney function is described on pp. 94–95) lie in the upper, posterior abdominal cavity on either side of the backbone. Each receives oxygen-rich blood through a renal artery, a branch of the aorta, and returns oxygen-poor (but 'filtered') blood along the renal vein to the inferior vena cava. The muscular bladder lies in the lower, pelvic region of the abdominal cavity. Each kidney is connected to the bladder by a ureter which opens in the inferior, posterior surface of the bladder. The inferior exit from the bladder is guarded by a sphincter muscle and leads to the urethra, which carries urine to the outside.*

ml (6–10 fl oz) of urine, the spinal cord sends impulses to the bladder that stimulate the bladder wall to contract, and the internal urethral sphincter to relax so that urine passes into the top of the urethra. Shortly after this, messages travelling up the spinal cord to the brain give the person a conscious awareness that their bladder is filling. During urination, or micturition, the external sphincter muscle is relaxed under conscious control and contraction of the bladder wall pushes urine out through the urethra. This conscious control is learnt during early childhood.

Water content

Water is vitally important to the body because it provides the medium inside cells in which the reactions of life take place and is a major component of extracellular fluids, such as tissue fluid and blood, that play a vital role in homeostasis by, for example, supplying oxygen, removing wastes and keeping cells warm. For example, the body of a young man of average body mass (about 70 kg/155 lb) will contain about 40 l (70 pt) of water, with about 25 l (45 pt) inside cells and 15 l (26 pt) in the form of extracellular fluid.

The amount of water in a human body depends on a person's age, sex and fat content. Adipose (fat) tissue contains less water than any other body tissue, including bone, so that the fatter a person is, the less water (in terms of percentage of body mass) she or he will contain (see table, above). Infants, with low bone and body fat masses, are about 70% water. Young males contain less water than infants, but more water than young females because of the latter's higher fat content. Older people of both sexes contain less water because as people age their fat content

WATER CONTENT	
Age/sex	Water content (% body mass)
Infant	72
Young man	59
Young woman	50
Older man/woman	45

increases. Regardless of the age, sex or fat content of the individual, it is essential to maintain stable water levels in both intracellular and extracellular 'compartments' of the body. Maintaining the water content at constant levels is one of the major roles of the kidneys.

Water balance

Every day, an average adult takes in about 2.5 l (4.5 pt) of water from both drinks and food as well as 'metabolic water' generated by aerobic cell respiration. Water is lost by sweating, in faeces, directly across the skin and from the lungs and in urine. While the table below shows the average amounts lost, the real proportions depend on how active a person is and the ambient temperature. Obviously, if someone sweats a lot, they will lose less water in their urine. This is mediated by the pituitary hormone ADH, the secretion of which increases if body fluids become more concentrated, thereby conserving water inside the body. This monitoring of the concentration of body fluids, particularly blood, is carried out by the hypothalamus. As well as causing the pituitary gland to release ADH should blood concentration increase, the hypothalamus also generates the conscious feeling of thirst, so that a person drinks water to dilute blood plasma. By varying the volume and concentration of urine released by the body, the kidneys ensure that daily water intake is balanced by daily water output.

WATER BALANCE			
Water intake		Water output	
Drinks	1,500 ml/2.6 pt	Urine	1,500 ml/2.6 pt
Food	750 ml/26 fl oz	Lost through skin and lungs*	700 ml/24.5 fl oz
Metabolic water	250 ml/8.75 fl oz	Sweat	200 ml/7 fl oz
		Faeces	100 ml/3.5 fl oz
Total	2,500 ml/4.4 pt	Total	2,500 ml/4.4 pt
* water vapour that passes out in exhaled air and water that is lost directly across the skin.			

MALE REPRODUCTIVE SYSTEM

Reproduction produces offspring by bringing together the DNA carried by male and female sex cells. Both male and female reproductive systems produce sex cells, but they have different constituent organs. The male reproductive system consists of two testes, the penis and the ducts and glands that link them.

Testes

From puberty, the testes manufacture sperm and secrete hormones, principally testosterone, that produce and maintain secondary sexual characteristics and stimulate sperm production. They hang outside the body in the scrotum: this ensures they are 3°C (5°F) below body temperature, which is ideal for sperm production. Each has 250–300 wedge-shaped lobules, each with 1–4 tightly coiled seminiferous tubules in which sperm are produced. Surrounding these are interstitial (Leydig) cells that release testosterone when stimulated by luteinizing hormone (LH) from the anterior pituitary gland. Testosterone and follicle stimulating hormone (FSH), another pituitary hormone, stimulate sperm production.

Sperm and spermatogenesis

With its long, streamlined shape a mature sperm is perfectly adapted to deliver a genetic payload to the female sex cell, the ovum. It is c.0.05 mm (0.002 in) long, with three functional areas: the head holds genetic material in the form of 23 chromosomes, the body has mitochondria that release energy for movement and the tail propels the sperm. A healthy, fertile male produces c.300 million mature sperm daily through spermatogenesis. Diploid stem cells called spermatogonia in the wall of the seminiferous tubule divide by mitosis to form primary spermatocytes which contains 46 chromosomes. These then divide by meiosis (see p. 111) to produce four immature haploid sperm cells, each containing 23 chromo-

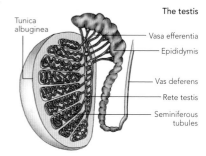

The testis

Tunica albuginea · Vasa efferentia · Epididymis · Vas deferens · Rete testis · Seminiferous tubules

somes. Immature sperm develop inside the tubule for 64 to 72 days before being pushed into the epididymis where they mature further – and gain motility – before entering the vas deferens. If sperm are not ejaculated they are reabsorbed as they age and their component are recycled.

Ducts and glands

A system of ducts (tubes) stores and transports sperm, while accessory glands that empty into the ducts produce fluids which activate and nurture sperm. The mixture of sperm and fluids is called semen.

• Epididymis

A highly coiled tube, c.6 m (20 ft) long, packed into a comma-shaped structure in which sperm mature, becoming capable of movement and of fertilizing an ovum.

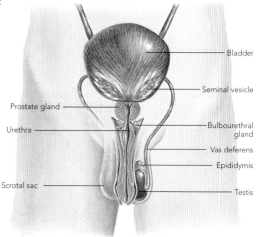

Male reproductive organs

Bladder · Seminal vesicle · Bulbourethral gland · Vas deferens · Epididymis · Testis

Prostate gland · Urethra · Scrotal sac

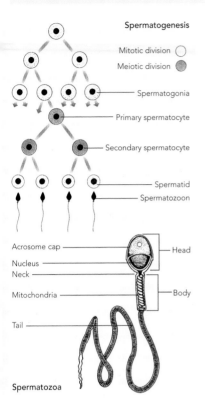

Spermatogenesis

Mitotic division ○
Meiotic division ●

Spermatogonia

Primary spermatocyte

Secondary spermatocyte

Spermatid
Spermatozoon

Acrosome cap — Head
Nucleus
Neck
Mitochondria — Body
Tail

Spermatozoa

• **Vas deferens**
Also called the ductus deferens, this is 45 cm (18 in) long and loops from the epididymis over the pubic bone, passing alongside the bladder before passing into the prostate gland and joining the urethra.

• **Seminal vesicles**
The seminal vesicles lie behind the bladder and each fuses with the end of its vas deferens. Fluid released by the seminal vesicle makes up c.60% of semen and contains both activating and fuel (fructose) chemicals. Seminal fluid is mixed with sperm as they are squeezed along the vas deferens just before ejaculation.

• **Prostate gland**
This chestnut-sized gland is just below the bladder surrounding the urethra where it leaves the bladder and the two vasa deferentia connect to it. Prostate secretions activate sperm, make up around 30% of the 3–5 ml (0.15–0.25 fl oz) of semen in each ejaculate and are mixed with sperm and seminal fluid during ejaculation.

• **Urethra**
The urethra runs along the lower side of the penis before opening at its tip. It carries urine and semen but not at the same time.

• **Bulbourethral glands**
Pea-sized glands that release a clear, alkaline secretion into the urethra during sexual arousal to neutralize its acidity, making it more 'sperm-friendly'.

Penis

This transfers semen into the female vagina during sexual intercourse. It consists of a root and a shaft which expands at its tip to form the glans covered by the foreskin (unless circumcised). The penis has three columns of spongy tissue: two corpora cavernosa (sing. corpus cavernosum) run in parallel along the upper part of the shaft; the corpus spongiosum runs along its underside, around the urethra, and forms the glans. During sexual arousal spaces within the spongy tissue fill with blood and make the normally limp penis erect.

Bladder (full)
Pubic bone
Prostate gland
Urethra
Corpus cavernosum
Epididymis
Testis
Corpus spongiosum

Seminal vesicle
Rectum
Bulbourethral gland
Anus
Vas deferens

FEMALE REPRODUCTIVE SYSTEM

The organs of the female reproductive system produce ova, the female sex cells; provide a location for the fertilization of an ovum by a sperm and, should fertilization occur, nurture and protect the developing fetus. The female reproductive system consists of the ovaries, fallopian tubes, uterus, vagina and external structures, known collectively as the vulva. Two pairs of labia, or vulval lips, form the sides of the vulva and surround and protect the entrance to the vagina and the clitoris. The clitoris is a small, sensitive erectile organ at the anterior end of the vulva.

Ovaries

Around 3 cm (1.2 in) long, the two almond-shaped ovaries make and release ova and secrete oestrogen and progesterone, sex hormones that control the menstrual cycle (see opposite) and develop and maintain secondary sexual characteristics such as breasts. Ova are produced by oogenesis, a process that takes years. At birth 2 million primary oocytes – immature ova, arrested in mid-meiosis – are present and they remain in 'suspended animation' until puberty, by when some 500,000 are still viable. Every month, from the first menstrual period, a small batch of oocytes starts to mature but only one completes meiosis to become a mature haploid ovum, containing 23 chromosomes, released during ovulation.

Fallopian tubes

The fallopian, or uterine, tubes are 10 cm (4 in) long and connect the ovaries to the uterus. At its ovarian end the tube expands to form finger-like fimbriae which form a funnel over the ovary but do not touch it. After ovulation, when an ovum bursts through the surface of the ovary, tiny hair-like cilia create a current that draws the ovum into the fallopian tube, through which it is carried to the uterus. If the ovum meets a sperm inside the fallopian tube and within 24 hours of ovulation, fertilization should occur.

Ovarian cycle This cross-section of the ovary shows an immature ovum (1) absorbing fluid and swelling into the sac-like Graafian follicle (2). As it reaches the surface (3), halfway through the menstrual cycle, the ovum bursts out into the peritoneal cavity to be collected by the fimbriae.
The empty follicular cyst then changes into the corpus luteum (4), which grows until menstruation, when it shrivels into a scab-like corpus albicans (5).

Uterus and vagina

The uterus (womb) is a small, pear-shaped, hollow organ that encloses, protects and nurtures the developing fetus in pregnancy. It has openings from the fallopian tubes

Female reproductive organs

Menstruation

Maturing Graafian follicle

Ovulation

Corpus luteum

Endometrium

Day 14 if pregnancy occurs

■ Oestrogen
■ Progesterone
■ FSH
■ LH
■ HCG

The menstrual cycle

Reproductive cycles

From puberty to menopause, a woman's reproductive system goes through a series of changes that lasts an average 28 days and prepares the body for possible pregnancy. Controlled by changing levels of hormones, these changes are caused by two closely linked reproductive cycles: the ovarian and menstrual cycles.

• Ovarian cycle

Inside one ovary each month several follicles, each containing an oocyte, start to enlarge. Just one becomes fully mature (a Graafian follicle) and bursts, releasing its ovum during ovulation around day 14 of the cycle. Follicle-stimulating hormone (FSH) from the pituitary gland causes an ovum to mature and stimulates follicles to release oestrogen. A sudden surge in levels of luteinizing hormone (LH), also from the pituitary gland, stimulates ovulation. The burst follicle forms a corpus luteum which releases progesterone.

• Menstrual cycle

During the menstrual cycle the endometrium thickens to receive an ovum if one is fertilized. At the start of the cycle the thickened lining from the last cycle is shed through the vagina during menstruation, or period. Then increasing levels of oestrogen produced by the ovary make the lining thicken once again. Increasing levels of progesterone following ovulation cause further thickening and vascularization. If, as normally happens, fertilization does not occur, the corpus luteum breaks down, oestrogen and progesterone levels drop and menstruation occurs. If fertilization occurs, the fertilized egg – now an embryo – implants in the endometrium and secretes human chorionic gonadotrophin (HCG) which maintains the corpus luteum and its progesterone production and, therefore, the integrity of the endometrium.

and opens through a channel in its cervix (neck) into the vagina. This muscular tube connects the uterus to the outside, accommodates the erect penis during sexual intercourse and forms the birth canal during childbirth. The uterine wall has a thick muscular layer, the myometrium, that stretches greatly in pregnancy and contracts to push the baby out during birth. Lining the uterine cavity is the endometrium, which undergoes a series of changes each month as part of the menstrual cycle.

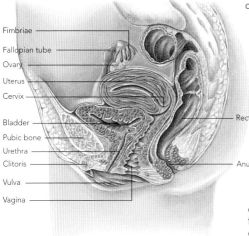

Fimbriae

Fallopian tube

Ovary

Uterus

Cervix

Bladder

Pubic bone

Urethra

Clitoris

Vulva

Vagina

Rectum

Anus

FERTILIZATION AND IMPLANTATION

Coitus

Coitus is the insertion of the erect penis into the vagina, followed by rhythmical movements ending in orgasm and the ejaculation of semen by the man. Initially sexual excitement is produced by sight, touch, sound and, perhaps, pheromones that stimulate smell. In the man, there is congestion of the corpora cavernosa and corpus spongiosum of the penis. In the woman, there is slight engorgement of the breasts and congestion of the clitoris and labia, with increased vaginal secretions. A prolonged phase of enjoyment can then follow when the penis is inserted into the vagina, provided the 'crescendo' to orgasm is controlled.

Orgasm is a series of rapid muscular contractions surrounding the male urethra that result in the ejaculation of the semen. This can be complemented by a simultaneous experience in the woman, in which the upper part of the vagina and a rhythmical 'sucking in' of the uterus draw the sperm to the right area. During sexual intercourse there are increases in blood pressure and rates of heartbeat and respiration. After orgasm there is physical relaxation.

Fertilization

The moment of conception is the most important stage of sexual reproduction. The joining of the two nuclei, each containing 23 chromosomes, to form a cell of 46 chromosomes, leads to the creation of an embryo.

The moment of conception

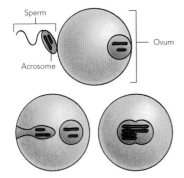

The sex of the baby is decided by the father's chromosomes – the XY sex pair. When the primary spermatocyte divides by meiosis to form the secondary spermatocytes, containing 23 chromosomes, either an X or a Y chromosome will move into each cell. The female pair of chromosomes are the same, XX, so all ova will contain the X chromosome. The fertilizing sperm will join the ova to form an XY male or XX female embryo. It is probable that there is less than 24 hours in which the ovum can be fertilized and, as the sperm survive for about 48 hours in the uterus and tubes, there is only a limited time each month during which conception is able to take place.

The sperm's journey to the ovum

The ejaculate of semen contains more than 350 million sperm. Ideally they are deposited adjacent to the cervix, where the vaginal enzymes dissolve the seminal mucus and release the sperm. They then swim into the cervical mucus, which is watery and soft enough at ovulation to allow many of the sperm to penetrate to the uterine cavity. Uterine contractions will then help them to move upwards to the fallopian tubes, where they again swim, perhaps with the help of the lining of ciliated cells, to reach the ovum at the mid-point of the tube. Only about 100 sperm survive the journey of nearly 24 hours and only one fertilizes the ovum. The ultimate fate of the surplus spermatozoa in the female genital tract is still not known.

The sperm's acrosome disappears as it dissolves the membrane of the ovum. The tail and body are shed when the head penetrates to join its 23 chromosomes with those of the ovarian nucleus.

Implantation of the ovum

It takes about a week for the fertilized ovum to pass down the fallopian tube and implant itself in the endometrium. The following description of implantation complements the diagram opposite.

Within hours of conception, mitosis begins with the development of a sphere of an increasing number of cells. The sphere starts as the blastomere (**1**), then becomes a morula (**2**) of about 64 cells. At this stage it changes into a hollow, fluid-containing ball – blastocyst (**3**) – with the inner cell mass at one end. It can now begin implantation (**4**) into the lining of the uterus. The outer ring of cells, now called the trophoblast, secretes enzymes that erode the endometrium. The trophoblastic cells spread into the endometrium, forming lacunae (fluid-bearing sacs) that penetrate the maternal circulation. This allows nutrition to take place. Ultimately, the trophoblast forms the outer layer of the placenta.

The inner cell mass splits into two layers: endoderm – ultimately the alimentary tract – which produces a yolk sac; and the ectoderm – ultimately the skin, brain and spinal cord – which produces the amniotic sac to surround and protect the embryo in a bag of fluid.

By the ninth day after conception, the blastocyst has sunk deep into the endometrium (**5**) and is already receiving nutrition from the mother. The trophoblast secretes human chorionic gonadotrophin (HCG) in order to maintain the progesterone production from the corpus luteum. This will continue until the end of the third month, when the placenta produces sufficient hormone to maintain this function until the end of pregnancy.

Implantation of the ovum

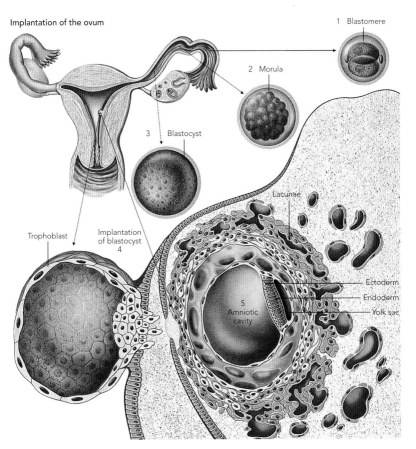

1 Blastomere

2 Morula

3 Blastocyst

Trophoblast

Implantation of blastocyst 4

Lacunae

Ectoderm

Endoderm

Yolk sac

5 Amniotic cavity

Growth of embryo

| Three-week embryo | Four-week embryo | Five-week embryo | Six-week embryo |

The first four weeks

The blastocyst begins to implant into the endometrium on the seventh day after conception. It consists of two distinct parts: a covering layer of the trophoblastic cells and an inner cell mass.

The trophoblast invades the maternal tissues and erodes the maternal blood vessels so that the surface is bathed in oxygen-carrying nutritious fluid. In addition the trophoblastic cells produce human chorionic gonadotrophin (HCG) to stimulate the production of progesterone and to help maintain pregnancy.

The inner cell mass develops a fluid-containing cavity from its upper surface (the amniotic sac), which eventually expands to line the inner surface of the trophoblastic cell layer. This layer ultimately forms the chorion of the fetal membranes and protects the embryo and fetus until parturition (childbirth).

The next two months

By the end of the third week (see artwork above), the mesodermal tissue begins to arrange itself into somites – a segmental arrangement that can be seen in humans in the ribs of the thoracic cage. Each somite of muscle is eventually supplied by its own blood vessels and nerves.

At four weeks, the embryo is 3 mm (0.125 in) long. It consists of 25 somites, the large bulge of the heart and has small ear pits in the head. It is not until the fifth week that a pair of pigmented discs appears on the head. These are the first signs of the eyes. In front is the small depression of the primitive nose. The limb buds, arms first and then legs, begin to grow by the sixth week.

At six weeks, the embryo has a tiny pulsating heart, 40 somites and miniature ear flaps. At this stage, the embryo is nearly 1.5 cm (0.5 in) long and the hands, fingers and feet are just about discernable.

Next, the somites lose their well-defined divisions and join up to form a solid mass of body tissue with recognizable thorax and abdomen and the beginnings of a neck. By the seventh week, the bulbous protuberance is clearly a head with well-defined nose, ears, eyes and mouth. The pelvis is starting to form and the end somites lose their tail-like appearance as the sacral bone is developed.

It is during this rapidly changing period, from the fourth to the seventh week, that congenital malformations may occur if the tissues fail to fold or divide correctly. External influences, such as disease or drugs, may damage the embryo.

By the eighth week, the embryo is approximately 2.5 cm (1 in) long and is recognizably human. It has distinct eyelids and separate fingers and its toes are developing.

From the end of the second month onwards, development is principally by growth and some alteration in proportion. By the end of 12 weeks, the embryo is

Seven-week
embryo

Eight-week
embryo or
fetus

5 cm (2 in) long and the mother's uterus is about the size of an orange. It is at this stage of development that the embryo is called a fetus.

The continuation of pregnancy

At the end of the fourth month, the fetus weighs about 125 g (4.5 oz) and is 12.5 cm (5 in) long. The genitalia are developing and ossification centres appear. The fetus is moving in the amniotic fluid and in the fifth month (see below left) the mother may feel these movements – known as 'quickening' – for the first time.

In the sixth month, the fetus starts to produce a layer of fat under the skin and a fine hair – called lanugo – that covers the head and body, which is also covered by a greasy substance – called vernix – that protects and lubricates the fetal skin, particularly during parturition. As the fetus grows, the proportion of amniotic fluid decreases. At 28 weeks, the fetus weighs about 500 g (17.5 oz) and its 140 heartbeats a minute can easily be heard; the fetus is now viable. Four to six weeks later, the head engages in the pelvis and remains there until parturition. During the last two months (see below right), it matures steadily and gains about 25 g (1 oz) in weight per day to reach about 3 kg (6.5 lb) at birth.

Five-month fetus

Nine-month fetus

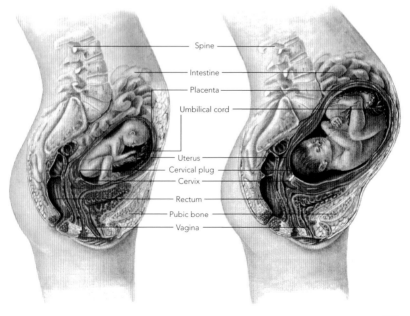

Spine
Intestine
Placenta
Umbilical cord
Uterus
Cervical plug
Cervix
Rectum
Pubic bone
Vagina

CHILDBIRTH

At about 280 days after conception, the fetus is expelled from the uterus. If pregnancy continues for too long the placenta begins to degenerate and the fetus is slowly starved of oxygen and nutrition.

Throughout pregnancy the uterine muscle has been contracting and relaxing. During the last few weeks, these contractions become stronger and are sometimes noticed by the mother. They help to keep the fetal head engaged in the pelvis (**A**). Labour is divided into three stages: the first is from the onset of labour, with regular rhythmical uterine contractions, to the moment when the cervix is fully dilated. This first stage may last from two to 24 hours or sometimes longer. The second stage is from the full dilation of the cervix to the moment of delivery and lasts less than two hours. The third stage is the expulsion of the placenta, cord and membranes. The placenta has to be carefully examined to make sure that parts of it have not been left behind which could cause a haemorrhage. The stages are described in greater detail below.

The first stage

The first stage starts with backache and regular uterine contractions that become gradually stronger and by the end occur about every two minutes, each lasting 30 to 40 seconds. As the head is forced deeper into the pelvis, it turns sideways (**B**) and the plug of cervical mucus is dislodged causing a 'show' of blood. The cervix is gradually stretched, thinned and dilated until it is wide enough (**C**) for the head to pass into the vagina. If it has not already done so, the amniotic sac ruptures.

The second and third stages

The second stage starts with the cervix fully dilated (**C**). The head moves deeper into the pelvis and turns again, so that the occiput is behind the symphysis pubis. The mother has a 'bearing down' sensation and can assist the powerful uterine contractions to force the fetus through the vagina. The vulva distends around the head and finally the baby is 'crowned' when the greatest circumference of the vulva is reached. The head extends (**D**) round the symphysis as it is

Sequence of normal birth

A

B

C

D

E

F

pushed out. The baby takes its first breath and lets out a cry. This expands the lungs and starts respiration, as well as obliterating the fetal circulation.

The baby can now be delivered (**E**) with the next contraction as the smaller shoulders and body easily follow the large head. At this moment the mother is usually given an injection of oxytocin and ergometrine to stimulate uterine contraction and the separation of the placenta.

The third stage follows 10 to 20 minutes later when the placenta has separated from the uterus and is expelled (**F**), along with the umbilical cord and membranes.

The puerperium

After parturition the uterus returns to normal size in about a month with loss of lochia, which is initially fresh blood later becoming creamy in colour. Menstruation will return in about two months unless suppressed by prolactin secretion during lactation. Excess body fluid and fat gradually disappear and softened ligaments regain their strength.

The baby is born with excess fluid, which it loses in the first few days, and a raised haemoglobin count level, which falls slowly with the appearance of slight jaundice. This is the result of raised levels of serum bilirubin from haemolysis and the immature liver's inability to excrete it.

Lactation

Throughout pregnancy the breasts have been enlarging under the stimulus of the anterior pituitary hormone, prolactin, to produce a watery milk (*see diagram, right*). In the last few weeks before parturition colostrum is produced and this is secreted for the first few days after birth. After this brief period, the mother's breasts begin to produce normal milk (**1**) and the baby's sucking (**2**) stimulates the hypothalamus. This continues the production of prolactin and also oxytocin from the posterior pituitary gland (**3**), which causes the breast alveoli to contract and force – 'let down' – the milk into the ducts (**4**).

Hormones in labour

● Progesterone
○ Oxytocin

Hormones in labour

The story of hormones in labour (*see diagram above*) is not fully understood. In some way their interreaction adjusts the actual onset of labour. Throughout the term of pregnancy, the production of progesterone makes the uterine muscle (**X**) relaxed and unresponsive to the posterior pituitary hormone – oxytocin. Toward the end of pregnancy, production of progesterone falls and there seems to be an increase in oestrogen. The combination of oxytocin and oestrogen initiates uterine contractions. The dilatation of the cervix (**Y**) increases oxytocin output and further reduces progesterone, so the contractions become stronger, longer and more frequent (**Z**). In the third stage, oxytocin helps to obliterate the spiral arteries in the uterine wall and initiate lactation. Oxytocin can be synthesized and is often used to start contraction of the uterus if labour is delayed.

Lactation

Colostrum

Milk

NEWBORN TO OLD AGE

Infancy

A newborn baby lies with its knees drawn up. It reflexly grasps any object that touches the palm and, when held upright, automatically steps as the feet touch something. It roots and sucks the nipple automatically. These reflexes disappear within a few weeks. At one month, the legs are straighter and by six weeks the head is lifted. The baby sleeps more often than not, but gradually the eyes move to focus on objects and, at about six weeks, smiling begins. By six months, the child's weight has doubled since birth and it sits unaided. At eight months, the preliminary gurglings of speech are heard and the thumb can be used. At about ten months, crawling starts. The child's weight has trebled since birth. The first step may be taken at age one. The first words may be spoken during the next two or three months.

Teeth

Deciduous teeth start to appear at about six months. By the age of three, the child has 20 teeth (see diagram below): eight incisors, four canines and eight premolars.

Between the ages of six and 12 years, the deciduous teeth are shed and replaced by the permanent dentition (see diagram, p. 85). A further six teeth, the molars, will appear in each jaw and by the age of 25, a total of 32 teeth will be present.

The tooth consists of three parts – the crown, neck and root. The **crown** consists of dense mineral (enamel) surrounding the hard dentine, which has a soft centre – the pulp. The pulp is filled with blood vessels, lymphatics and the nerve, which reach it through the root canal. The **neck** of a tooth adheres to the gum, while the **root** penetrates the bone, where it is held in place by a ligament and cementum.

▲ *Milk teeth By the age of three, a child has 20 'milk' teeth – eight incisors, four canines and eight premolars.*

Puberty

Puberty is the moment when sexual maturation has reached the point where sexual reproduction is possible. A period of development around puberty takes about two years and will usually start earlier in girls than it does in boys.

In girls, between the ages of 10 and 16, there are changes in the subcutaneous fat – hips and shoulders become more rounded, the breasts develop and the pubic and axillary hair grows. The first menstruation – menarche – establishes a definite point of maturity.

In boys, between the ages of 12 and 17, the shoulders broaden, the muscles strengthen and the genitalia develop and darken to become covered with pubic hair. The larynx lengthens and the voice 'breaks' to become deeper. Spontaneous erections occur and the nocturnal emissions of sperm are perhaps less dramatic a sign of sexual maturity than the menarche.

Adolescence

Adolescence is a time of great physical and emotional change and can cause anxiety without the appropriate care and guidance. It is a time when social, intellectual and sexual interests expand and broaden. Adolescents may experiment with different lifestyles and identities. The young person is no longer a child. She or he is more or less physiologically mature, but may feel frustrated by the constraints on her or his freedom in comparison with adults.

The intense emotions of adolescence can be expressed by the individual in a number of different ways, mostly harmless. However, adolescents often experience dramatic moodswings. Periods of great enthusiasm may be followed by periods of almost depressive lethargy.

The young adult

As the turmoil of adolescence settles, young adults (18–26) are believed to be at their physical prime. In addition to body maturity, relationships with family and society may be more positive and there is generally a greater awareness and control of emotions and sexual desire. The first tentative adolescent meetings with the opposite sex have passed and mature relationships develop. Entrance into the world of work may provide an element of independence and many young adults may find greater self-confidence.

Middle age

The most stable period of life is usually considered to start around the age of 30. It can be a time of relative financial and emotional security with greater emphasis placed on relationships. Sexual desire is less urgent but often more satisfactory and women are considered to be at their sexual peak.

In women, the menopause – the final cessation of menstruation – generally starts around the age of 50. It may be followed by a time of hormonal disturbance leading to hot flushes, tensions and sometimes depression. A programme of hormone replacement treatment (HRT) can help to ease many of the problems that accompany the menopause.

Although physical health usually remains good, there is a tendency to gain weight, accompanied by a slight, but definite loss of athletic skills. Men may begin to experience hair loss. In the later years there is an increase in the death rate, particularly from heart disease and cancer of the lungs.

Old age and senescence

The definition of 'old age' varies from society to society and also between individuals. In a general manner, however, it can be characterized by changes in close familial relationships, financial status and personal health. Common health issues include arthritis and a gradual loss of visual acuity and hearing, which may lead to a slower reaction time.

As we age, the adrenal glands continue to secrete sex hormones and the slight androgenic effect may produce slight hair loss in women, while in men there may be the oestrogen effect of female fat distribution and less beard growth. Cancer and other illnesses are common and often fatal.

Senescence is the period of real ageing and may begin long before or long after the arbitrary point of 'old age'. The skin loses its elasticity and gains wrinkles. The hair loses its colour, becoming white as it fills with microscopic bubbles of air. The senses of vision, hearing and taste deteriorate. The joints become rough and arthritic, while the muscles weaken. The bones in the skeleton soften as the structure deteriorates and calcium is removed, causing the bent spine of many of the elderly.

The nervous system begins to lose nerve cells, leading to failure of memory – initially for recent events but later a gradual dementia may occur. The cerebellum is affected, producing a loss of co-ordination, tremor of the hands and hesitation in speech. The heat centre in the thalamus is less responsive and a cold environment may cause a drop in body temperature, a condition known as hypothermia, that can lead to coma and death. Deterioration in the heart and lungs may cause irregularities of cardiac rhythm and often breathlessness.

In some people these ageing processes may take place faster in one system than another. This can be seen with dementia occurring while the body is fit or osteoarthritis crippling an otherwise perfectly healthy person.

In some cases, the pressures of senescence are enormous and the individual may need professional help. In extreme cases, admission to hospital is the only way of giving sufficient basic nursing care.

▶ *Four female generations of a family*, from the great-grandmother at far right to great-granddaughter at far left.

GENES AND INHERITANCE

Our identity depends on the genetic material we inherit from our parents. Inside the nucleus of most of our body cells (apart from sex cells) is a set of instructions for building a human being. The instructions, called genes, are contained in 23 pairs of chromosomes constructed from DNA (deoxyribonucleic acid). All the DNA in one set of chromosomes is called a genome. By 2003 the Human Genome Project had completely analysed the DNA in human chromosomes and showed there are around 25,000 genes in one genome.

The 23 chromosome pairs are matched (homologous): one member of each pair is from the mother and one from the father. Members of each pair carry the same genes in the same locations. While each gene controls a particular characteristic, it may have different alleles or forms. When two different alleles of a particular gene

exist in a cell only one, the dominant allele, produces any effect: the other recessive (hidden) allele is inactive, although it may be passed on to the next generation. Identical alleles on homologous chromosomes are called homozygous: where they are different they are called heterozygous.

Many aspects of inheritance depend on chance events. Sex cells (gametes), produced by meiosis (see opposite), contain just one set of chromosomes derived randomly from the parental sets. When sperm and ovum meet at fertilization, the resulting human has a unique genetic identity (except for identical twins). That person's features are determined not by a 'blending' of maternal and paternal genes but by the expression of dominant genes. In addition, a person's gender depends purely on whether an X- or a Y-chromosome-carrying sperm fertilizes the ovum.

Twin births

A
Single ovum

Single placenta

Identical twins

B
Two ova

Two placentae

Fraternal twins

▲ *Sex determination*
A pair of chromosomes –
X (red) and Y (black) –
determines sex. Female
body cells contain two
matching X chromosomes
(XX). So an ovum produced
by meiosis can only contain
an X chromosome. Male
body cells contain one X and
one Y chromosome (XY) so a
sperm can contain either X
or Y chromosome. An ovum
fertilized by a Y-carrying
sperm produces a male: one
fertilized by an X-carrying
sperm produces a female.

Twins Twin births occur about once in every 70 pregnancies. Identical twins (**A**) are always the same sex, developing from mitotic division of the same fertilized ovum. Each fetus has its own amniotic sac,

but they share a single placenta. Fraternal, non-identical twins (**B**), develop from two separate ova that have been fertilized at the same time by different spermatozoa. They have separate placentae.

Meiosis and gamete formation

Most body cells divide by a process called mitosis (see p. 9) which results in two identical 'daughter' cells that are diploid (contain two sets of 23 chromosomes). Meiosis, on the other hand, is a form of cell division that takes place only in the ovaries and testes and produces the gametes (sex cells) – ova or sperm. Gametes are haploid (have one set of 23 chromosomes) and differ from each other and from their diploid 'parent'. When gametes fuse at fertilization the resulting zygote has a full set of genetic instructions to 'build' a new person who will share many characteristics of her or his parents but will be genetically unique. Occasionally more or fewer than 46 chromosomes are present, generally resulting in the non-viability of the embryo, but in some cases – as with Down's syndrome, where there is an extra copy of chromosome 21 – a baby can develop and survive.

Meiosis (right) has two phases, I and II. For simplicity only four chromosomes are shown here, i.e. two pairs of homologous chromosomes with, in each pair, one maternal (red) and one paternal (black).

• Meiosis I

At the start of meiosis (and mitosis) long chromatin (DNA) strands in the nucleus of a gamete-producing cell (spermatocyte or oocyte) condense to form chromosomes (1), each of which replicates itself (2) so it consists of two identical linked strands (chromatids). Homologous chromosomes lie close to each other and randomly swap sections of their chromatids (3): this gene swapping is called crossing over and it contributes to the gametes' genetic variety. Now the homologous pairs line up across the equator (centre) of the cell (4) then separate and move to opposite poles (ends) of the cell (5) which now divides.

• Meiosis II

The two haploid daughter cells (6) undergo a mitosis-like division with the chromosomes lining up on their equators (7). The chromosomes split with 'sister' chromatids (now called chromosomes) migrating to opposite poles (8) of the cell, which divides. The resulting gametes (9) are haploid and not identical; whether a gamete receives the maternal or paternal member of a homologous pair is a matter of chance.

▲ *Inheritance of eye colour* Blue and brown eye colours are controlled by two alleles: the 'brown' allele' is dominant. Where the brown-eyed parent is homozygous for the brown allele and the blue-eyed parent is homozygous for the blue allele (**A**), their children can have only brown eyes. But if both brown-eyed parents are heterozygous for both alleles (**B**) they have a one in four chance of a blue-eyed child at any one conception.

Meiosis – gamete formation

Chromosomes crossing over

111

A

an induced abortion is up to 24 weeks after conception.

abscess Collection of pus anywhere in the body, contained in a cavity of inflamed tissue. It is caused by bacterial infection.

acidosis Abnormal condition in which the acidity of the body tissues and fluids is unduly high. It may arise in a number of conditions, including kidney failure, severe diabetes, shock and some forms of poisoning. Symptoms include breathlessness, weakness and general malaise.

abortion Termination of pregnancy before a fetus is sufficiently advanced to survive outside the mother's uterus. **Spontaneous** abortion, better known as a miscarriage, occurs in c.20% of apparently normal pregnancies. Miscarriages in the first three months of pregnancy are usually caused by fetal abnormalities. Miscarriages later in pregnancy may be caused by defects in the maternal environment, such as reproductive system disorders. Induced or therapeutic abortion is the termination of pregnancy by drugs or surgery. The rights of the fetus and the mother's right to choose provoke much political and ethical debate. Currently, the legal time limit in the UK for

acne Inflammatory disorder of the sebaceous (oil-producing) glands of the skin resulting in skin eruptions such as blackheads and infected spots; it is seen mostly on the face, neck and back. Acne is common in both sexes at puberty. It does not usually persist beyond early adulthood. Severe cases can be treated with drugs.

acquired immune deficiency syndrome (AIDS) Potentially fatal disease caused by a retrovirus, called HUMAN IMMUNODEFICIENCY VIRUS (HIV), that mainly attacks T-4 cells (which help the production of antibodies) and renders the body's immune system incapable of resisting infection.

◄ *AIDS The sequence of false-colour TEMs shows the formation of an HIV particle at the surface of an infected lymphocyte. The first appearance of the virus (top left) is as a small bump (red) on the surface of the cell. The virus then buds out (top right) and is eventually cut off from the cell membrane.*
The newly released virus particle (bottom left) has an outer shell of dense material (red) which is reorganized to form the central nucleoid that becomes characteristically elongated in the mature virus (bottom right). Magnification: ×100,000.

A

► *Acupuncture Model of a man's head marked with a acupuncture chart. Meridians (lines) and points are mapped out across the skin. The meridians relate to channels of energy within the body. Imbalances in the flow of energy are thought to cause pain and disease. The insertion of needles at precise points (marked by dots), at different angles, temperatures and speeds according to the disorder, is thought to stimulate energy flow. Acupuncture may work by inducing the production of natural analgesics within the central nervous system or by stimulating nerves which inhibit the original pain.*

The first diagnosis was made in New York in 1979. In 1983, scientists at the Pasteur Institute in France and the National Cancer Institute in the USA isolated HIV as the cause of the disease. The virus can remain dormant in infected cells for up to ten years. Initial **AIDS-related complex (ARC)** symptoms include severe weight loss and fatigue. The infection may develop into the AIDS syndrome, characterized by secondary infections, neurological damage and cancers. AIDS is transmitted only by a direct exchange of body fluids. Transmission is most commonly through sexual intercourse, the sharing of contaminated needles by intravenous drug users and the uteri of infected mothers to their babies. In the United States and Europe, more than 65% of victims have been homosexual or bisexual men. However, 90% of reported cases are in the developing world and many victims are heterosexual. AIDS is now the leading cause of death in sub-Saharan Africa. Recent combinations of drugs have met with some success in controlling symptoms. By 2006, *c.*25 million people had died from AIDS.

acupuncture System of medical treatment in which long needles are inserted into the body to assist healing or relieve pain, or for anaesthetic purposes. In ancient Chinese philosophy, acupuncture is proposed to restore the balance of yin and yang by freeing the flow of life energy (chi) through pathways in the body. A possible scientific explanation is that the needles activate deep sensory nerves that stimulate the pituitary gland and hypothalamus to produce endorphins.

addiction Inability to control the use of a particular substance, resulting in physiological or psychological dependence. It is most frequently associated with drug addiction. In a medical context, addiction requires a physical dependence. When the dose of a drug is reduced or withdrawn, the addict experiences withdrawal syndromes. Psychological dependence on activities such as gambling or exercise is difficult to distinguish from a disorder or mania.

adhesion In medicine, fibrous band of connective tissue developing at a site of inflammation or damage: it may bind together adjacent tissues, such as loops of intestine, occasionally causing obstruction. Most adhesions result from inflammation or surgery.

◄ *Albino* A male and female both carrying a recessive gene (green) for albinism (**A**) have a 75% chance of having a normal child (**B**, **D** or **E**) and 25% of an albino child (**C**). The normal gene (orange or purple) in both produces normal skin colour. This is due to an amino acid, phenylalanine (**1**), which has been converted to tyrosine (**2**) and then to melanin (**3**). A recessive gene in double quantity only allows the conversion of phenylalanine to tyrosine (**F**) resulting in an albino with a lack of pigment in the skin, hair and eyes.

adrenaline Hormone secreted by the adrenal glands (*see* p. 57), important in preparing the body's response to stress. It has widespread effects in the body, increasing the strength and rate of heartbeat and the rate and depth of breathing, diverting blood from the skin and digestive system to the heart and muscles, and stimulating the release of glucose from the liver to increase energy supply by promoting increased respiration. Synthetic adrenaline is used medicinally in the resuscitation of patients in shock or following cardiac arrest.

agglutination Clumping of BACTERIA or ERYTHROCYTES by antibodies that react with ANTIGENS on the cell surface.

AIDS *See* ACQUIRED IMMUNE DEFICIENCY SYNDROME (AIDS)

albino Person or animal with a rare hereditary absence of pigment from the skin, hair and eyes. The hair is white and the skin and eyes are pink because, in the absence of pigment, the blood vessels are visible. The eyes are abnormally sensitive to light and vision is often poor.

albumin (albumen) Type of water-soluble protein occurring in animal tissues and fluids. Principal forms are egg albumin (egg white) and milk and blood albumins.

allergy Disorder caused by an overreaction of the body's immune system as a result of hypersensitivity to a normally harmless substance, termed an allergen. Some 25% of people suffer from allergies. Common allergens include pollen, dust, pet hairs, wasp stings, medicines and foods such as peanuts. The immune system releases IgE antibodies that stimulate mast cells to release histamine, which causes an unnecessary inflammatory response in the affect area. Typical reactions include itchy eyes, runny nose and sneezing (HAY FEVER); 'wheezing' and difficulty breathing (ASTHMA) or skin eruptions and itching (ECZEMA). In a few cases life-threatening anaphylactic shock and death may result. A tendency to allergic reactions is often hereditary.

Alzheimer's disease Degenerative condition characterized by memory loss and progressive mental impairment: it is the most common cause of DEMENTIA. Sometimes seen in middle age, Alzheimer's becomes increasingly common with advancing age. Many factors have been implicated, but the precise cause is unknown.

American Medical Association (AMA) US federation of 54 state and territorial medical associations founded in 1847. The AMA develops programmes to provide scientific information for the profession and healtheducation materials for the public. In 2003, over 260,000 physicians were members.

amphetamine DRUG that stimulate the central nervous system. These drugs (also known as 'pep pills' or 'speed') can lead to drug abuse and dependence. They can induce a temporary sense of well-being, often followed by fatigue and depression. *See also* ADDICTION

amylase Digestive enzyme secreted by the salivary glands (salivary amylase) and the pancreas (pancreatic amylase). It aids digestion by breaking down starch into maltose (a disaccharide) and then glucose (a monosaccharide).

anabolic steroid Any of a group of hormones that stimulate the growth of tissue. Synthetic versions are used in medicine to treat OSTEOPOROSIS and some types of ANAEMIA: they may also be prescribed to aid weight gain in severely ill or elderly patients. These drugs are associated with a number of side-effects, including acne, fluid retention, liver damage and masculinization in women. Some athletes have been known to abuse anabolic steroids in order to increase muscle bulk.

anaemia Condition in which there is a shortage of haemoglobin, the oxygen-carrying pigment contained in erythrocytes (red blood cells). Symptoms include weakness, pallor, breathlessness, faintness, palpitations and lowered resistance to infection. It may be due to a decrease in the production of haemoglobin or red blood cells, excessive destruction of red blood cells or blood loss. Worldwide, iron deficiency is the commonest cause of anaemia.

anaesthesia State of insensibility or loss of sensation produced by disease or by various anaesthetic drugs used during surgical procedures. During **general** (or total) anaesthesia, the entire human body becomes insensible and the individual sleeps. In **local** anaesthesia only a specific part of the body is rendered insensible, and the patient remains conscious. A general anaesthetic may be either an injected drug, such as the BARBITURATE **thiopentone**, used to induce unconsciousness, or an inhalation agent such as **halothane**, which is used to maintain anaesthesia for surgery. Local anaesthetics, such as **lignocaine**, numb the relevant part of the body by blocking the transmission of impulses through the sensory nerves which supply it.

analgesic DRUG that relieves or prevents pain without causing loss of consciousness.

▶ *Alzheimer's disease*
Computer graphic of a vertical (coronal) slice through the brain of a patient with Alzheimer's disease (left) compared with a normal brain (right). The brain of the Alzheimer's patient has shrunk due to the degeneration and death of nerve cells. Apart from a decrease in brain volume, the surface of the brain is often more deeply folded. Alzheimer's accounts for most cases of senile dementia. Symptoms include memory loss, disorientation and delusion.

115

A

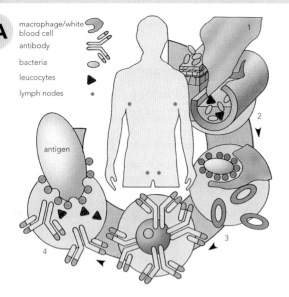

macrophage/white blood cell
antibody
bacteria
leucocytes
lymph nodes
antigen

◄ *Antibody* When bacteria enter the blood stream at the site of a wound (*1*), macrophages (white blood cells) engulf some (*2*) and carry them to the lymph nodes (*3*) where B-cells (blue) produce antibodies to bind with the unique antigen proteins on the surface of the invading bacteria (*4*). When the antibodies released into the blood stream attach themselves to the bacteria they stimulate certain leucocytes to destroy them.

It does not cure the cause of the pain, but helps to deaden the sensation. Some analgesics are also NARCOTICS. Many have valuable anti-inflammatory properties. Common analgesics include aspirin, codeine and morphine. *See also* ANAESTHESIA

androgen General name for male sex hormones, such as TESTOSTERONE.

anemia *See* ANAEMIA

angina Pain in the chest due to an insufficient blood supply to the heart, usually associated with diseased coronary arteries. Generally induced by exertion or stress, it is treated with drugs, such as glyceryl trinitrate, or by surgery.

anorexia nervosa Abnormal loss of the desire to eat. A pathological condition, it is seen mainly in young women anxious to lose weight. It can result in severe emaciation and in rare cases may be life-threatening. *See also* BULIMIA NERVOSA

anthrax Contagious disease, chiefly of livestock, caused by the microbe *Bacillus anthracis*. Human beings can catch anthrax from contact with infected

animals or their hides. In 2001, five US citizens died after contact with mail contaminated by anthrax spores, provoking worries of bio-terrorism.

antibiotic Substance that is capable of stopping the growth of, or destroying, BACTERIA and other microorganisms. Antibiotics are germicides that are safe enough to be eaten or injected into the body. The post-1945 introduction of antibiotics revolutionized medical science, making possible the virtual elimination of once widespread and often fatal diseases, such as TYPHOID FEVER, PLAGUE and CHOLERA. Some antibiotics are selective – that is, they are effective against specific microorganisms. Those effective against a large number of microorganisms are known as **broad-spectrum** antibiotics. Important antibiotics include PENICILLIN, the first widely used antibiotic, streptomycin and the tetracyclines. Some bacteria have developed ANTIBIOTIC RESISTANCE. *See also* ANTISEPTIC

antibiotic resistance Resistance to antibiotic drugs acquired by many BACTERIA and other pathogens (disease-causing microorganisms). Because some bacteria survive while non-resistant strains die, they pass their resistance to their progeny and resistance increases in the population. Some bacteria have the ability to pass the genes for antibiotic resistance to other organisms of different species on plasmids (small lengths of DNA). Spread of resistance is accelerated by routine prescription of antibiotics to humans and unregulated application to farm animals for the purpose of disease prevention rather than cure. An inadequate dose or failure to complete a course of antibiotics increases the chances of resistant microorganisms surviving to breed. This may lead to the return of epidemics of untreatable infectious disease.

antibody Protein synthesized in the BLOOD in response to the entry of 'foreign' substances or organisms into the body. Each episode of bacterial or viral infection prompts the production of a specific antibody to fight the disease. After the infection has cleared, the antibody remains in the blood to fight off any future invasion.

antigen Substance or organism that induces the production of an ANTIBODY, part of the body's defence mechanism against disease. An antibody reacts specifically with the antigen.

antihistamine Any one of certain drugs that counteracts or otherwise prevents the effects of histamine, a natural substance released by the body in response

to injury, or more often as part of an allergic reaction. Histamine can produce symptoms such as sneezing, running nose and burning eyes. *See also* HAY FEVER

antiseptic Chemicals that destroy or stop the growth of many microorganisms. Antiseptics are weak germicides that can be used on the skin. The English surgeon Joseph Lister pioneered the use of antiseptics in 1867. One commonly used is alcohol. *See also* ANTIBIOTIC

antitoxin ANTIBODY produced by the body in response to a TOXIN. It is specific in action and neutralizes the toxin. Antitoxin sera are used to treat and prevent bacterial diseases such as TETANUS and DIPHTHERIA.

aphasia Group of disorders of language arising from disease of or damage to the brain. In aphasia, a person has problems formulating or comprehending speech and difficulty in reading and writing.

appendicitis Inflammation of the appendix caused by obstruction and infection. Symptoms include severe pain in the central abdomen, nausea and vomiting. Acute appendicitis is generally treated by surgery. A ruptured appendix can cause peritonitis and even death.

arteriosclerosis Blanket term for degenerative diseases of the arteries, in partic-

▶ *Anthrax False-colour SEM of spores of the rod-shaped bacteria* Bacillus anthracis, *the causative agent of anthrax in farm animals. The disease is transmitted to man by contact with infected animal hair, excrement or hides. Bacilli attack either the lungs, causing pneumonia, or the skin, producing severe ulceration (malignant pustule). In the body the bacteria appear singly or in pairs, but when cultured they link up, as seen here. Magnification: ×2,825.*

A

◀ **Arthritis** *In rheumatoid arthritis (A) the synovial membrane (1) becomes inflamed and thickened and produces increased synovial fluid within the joint (2). The capsule and surrounding tissues (3) become inflamed, while joint cartilage is damaged (4). Peripheral joints are usually affected. Blood tests show rheumatoid factor. Osteoarthritis (B), a degenerative disease, involves thinning of cartilage (5), loss of joint space (6) and bone damage (7). Heavily used or weight-bearing joints are affected. Blood tests are normal.*

ular **atherosclerosis** (hardening of the arteries). It is caused by deposits of fatty materials and scar tissue on the artery walls, which narrow the channel and restrict blood flow, causing an increased risk of heart disease, stroke or gangrene. Evidence suggests that predisposition to the disease is hereditary. Risk factors include smoking, inactivity, obesity and a diet rich in animal fats and refined sugar. Treatment is by drugs and, in some instances, surgery to replace a diseased length of artery.

arthritis Inflammation of the joints, with pain and restricted mobility. The most common forms are osteoarthritis and rheumatoid arthritis. **Osteoarthritis**, common among the elderly, occurs with erosion of joint cartilage and degenerative changes in the underlying bone. It is treated with ANAL-GESICS and anti-inflammatories and, in some cases (especially a diseased hip), by joint replacement surgery. **Rheumatoid arthritis**, more common in women, is generally more disabling. It is an autoimmune disease which may disappear of its own accord but is usually slowly progressive. Treatment includes analgesics to relieve pain. The most severe cases may need to be treated with CORTISONE injections, drugs to suppress immune activity or joint replacement surgery. *See also* RHEUMATISM

artificial insemination Method of inducing PREGNANCY without sexual intercourse by injecting sperm into the female genital tract. Artificial insemination is increasingly used to enable women without a male partner to have children. *See also* IN VITRO FERTILIZATION (IVF)

asthma Disorder of the respiratory system in which the bronchi (air passages) of the lungs go into spasm, making breathing difficult. It can be triggered by infection, air pollution, allergy, certain drugs, exertion or emotional stress. **Allergic** asthma may be treated by injections aimed at lessening sensitivity to specific allergens. Otherwise treatment is with bronchodilators to relax the bronchial muscles and ease breathing. In severe asthma, inhaled steroids may be given. Children often outgrow asthma, while some people suddenly acquire the disease in middle age. Air pollution is increasing the number of asthma sufferers. *See also* BRONCHITIS; EMPHYSEMA

astigmatism Defect of vision in which the curvature of the lens differs from one perpendicular plane to another. It can be compensated for by corrective lenses.

ataxia Condition where muscles are uncoordinated. It results in clumsiness, irregular and uncontrolled movements and difficulties with speech. It may be caused by physical injury to the brain or nervous system, by a STROKE, or by disease.

atrophy Shrinking or wastage of tissues or organs. It may be associated with disease, malnutrition or, in the case of muscle atrophy, with disuse.

atropine Poisonous alkaloid drug ($C_{17}H_{23}NO_3N$) obtained from certain plants such as *Atropa belladonna* (deadly nightshade). Atropine is used medicinally to regularize the heartbeat during anaesthesia, to dilate the pupil of the eye and to treat motion sickness.

autism Disorder, usually first appearing in early childhood, characterized by a withdrawal from social behaviour, communication difficulties and ritualistic behaviour. Autistic people have difficulty understanding themselves or others as agents with varying beliefs and desires. The causes of autism may originate in genetics, brain damage or psychology.

autoimmune disease Any one of a group of disorders caused by the body's production of antibodies which attack the body's own tissues. One example of such an autoimmune disease is systemic LUPUS ERYTHEMATOSUS (SLE), an inflammation of the connective tissue occurring most often in young women. The occasional presence of so-called auto-antibodies in an individual does not necessarily indicate autoimmune disease.

Ayurveda System of medicine practised by the ancient Hindus and derived from the Vedas (ancient, most sacred writings of Hinduism). It is still practised in India.

bacillus Genus of rod-like BACTERIA that is present everywhere in the air and soil. One example of a species that is pathogenic in man is *Bacillus anthracis*, which causes ANTHRAX.

▶ *Bacteria occur in spherical forms called cocci (A), rod-like bacilli (B), and spiral spirilla (C). Cocci occur in clumps, e.g. staphylococci (1), pairs called diplococci (2) or chains, e.g. streptococci (3). Unlike cocci, bacilli are mobile: some are termed peritrichous and use flagella (4) to swim, while other monotrichous forms use a single flagellum (5). Bacilli can also form spores (6) to survive harsh conditions. Spirilla may be either cork-screw-shaped spirochaetes, like Leptospira (7), or less coiled and flagellated, such as Spirillum (8)*

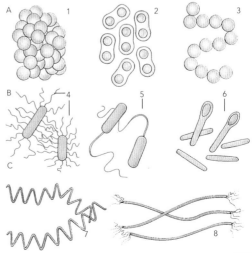

119

B

bacteria Simple, unicellular, prokaryotic organisms. They lack a clearly defined nucleus and organelles. Many are motile, swimming by means of whip-like flagella. In adverse conditions, many can remain dormant inside highly resistant spores with thick protective coverings. Although pathogenic bacteria are a major cause of human disease, many bacteria are harmless or even beneficial to humans by providing an important link in food chains, by decomposing plant and animal tissue or converting free nitrogen and sulphur into amino acids and other compounds that plants and animals can use. Most bacteria belong to the kingdom Eubacteria. *See picture*, p. 119

bacteriology Scientific study of BACTERIA. Bacteria were first observed in the 17th century by Anton van Leeuwenhoek, but it was not until the researches of Louis Pasteur and Robert Koch in the mid-19th century that bacteriology was established as a scientific discipline.

bacteriophage VIRUS that lives on and infects BACTERIA. It has a protein head containing a core of DNA and a protein tail. Discovered in 1915, it is important in the study of genetics.

barbiturate DRUG used as a sedative or to induce sleep. Highly addictive and dangerous in high doses, or in combination with other drugs such as alcohol or TRANQUILLIZERS, most barbiturates are no longer prescribed. **Short-acting** barbiturates are used in surgery to induce general ANAESTHESIA. **Long-acting** formulations are prescribed for epilepsy.

basal metabolic rate (BMR) Minimum amount of energy required by the body to sustain basic life processes, including breathing, circulation and tissue repair. It is calculated by measuring oxygen consumption. Metabolic rate increases above BMR during physical activity or fever, or under the influence of some drugs (including caffeine). It falls below the basal metabolic rate during sleep, general ANAESTHESIA or starvation. BMR is highest in children and decreases with age. *See also* METABOLISM

BCG (**B**acille **C**almette **G**uérin) Vaccine against TUBERCULOSIS. It was discovered by the French bacteriologists Albert Calmette (1863–1933) and Camille Guérin (1872–1961).

Bell's palsy Paralysis of a facial nerve causing weakness of the muscles on one side of the face. The condition, which may be due to viral infection, usually disappears spontaneously or may be treated with drugs or, rarely, surgery.

◄ *Beta-blocker* Polarized light micrograph (PLM) of crystals of the beta-blocker drug Propranolol (Propranolol hydrochloride). Beta-blocker drugs selectively block receptors of the sympathetic nervous system in heart muscle, in the process decreasing the activity of the heart. Propranolol may also be used to treat an overactive thyroid gland and to prevent migraine. Magnification: ×312.

bends (decompression sickness) Syndrome, mostly seen in divers, featuring pain in the joints, dizziness, nausea and paralysis. It is caused by the release of nitrogen into the tissues and blood. This occurs if there is a too rapid a return to normal atmospheric pressure after a period of breathing high-pressure air (when the body absorbs more nitrogen). Treatment involves gradual decompression in a hyperbaric chamber.

benzodiazepine Any of a group of mood-altering drugs, such as **librium** and **valium**, that are used primarily to treat severe anxiety or insomnia. They intervene in the transmission of nerve signals in the central nervous system and were originally developed as muscle relaxants. Today, they are the most widely prescribed TRANQUILLIZERS. *See* **nervous system**, pp. 34–55

beriberi Disease caused by a deficiency of vitamin B$_1$ (thiamine) and other vitamins in the diet. Symptoms include weakness, OEDEMA (waterlogging of the tissues) and degeneration of nerves. The disease is rare in the developed world.

beta-blocker Any of a class of DRUGS that block impulses to beta nerve receptors in various tissues throughout the body, including the heart, airways and peripheral arteries. These drugs are mainly prescribed to regulate the heartbeat, reduce blood pressure and relieve ANGINA. They are also being used in an increasingly wide range of other conditions, including GLAUCOMA, liver disease, thyrotoxicosis, MIGRAINE and anxiety states. Beta-blockers are not suitable for patients with asthma or severe lung disease.

bile Bitter yellow, brown or green alkaline fluid secreted by the liver and stored in the gall bladder. Important in digestion, it enters the duodenum via the bile duct. Its bile salts emulsify fats (allowing easier digestion and absorption) and neutralize stomach acids. *See* pp. 89–93

bioengineering Application of engineering techniques to medical and biological problems such as devices to aid or replace defective or inadequate body organs, as in the production of artificial limbs and hearing aids.

biofeedback In alternative medicine, the use of monitoring systems to provide information about body processes to enable them to be controlled voluntarily. By observing data on events that are normally involuntary, such as breathing and the heartbeat, many people learn to gain control over them to some extent in order to improve their sense of well-being. The technique has proved helpful in a number of conditions, including MIGRAINE and HYPERTENSION.

biopsy Removal of a small piece of tissue from a patient for examination for evidence of disease. An example is the CERVICAL SMEAR (pap test), performed in order to screen for possible pre-cancerous changes that can lead to cervical cancer.

biotechnology Use of biological processes for medical, industrial or manufacturing purposes. Humans have long used yeast for brewing and bacteria for products such as cheese and yoghurt. Biotechnology now enjoys a wider application. By growing microorganisms in the laboratory, new drugs and chemicals are produced. Genetic engineering techniques of cloning, splicing and mixing genes facilitate, for example, growing crops outside their normal environment and vaccines that fight specific diseases. Hormones are also produced, such as insulin for treating diabetes.

bipolar disorder *See* MANIC DEPRESSION

birth, Caesarean Delivery of a baby by a surgical incision made through the abdomen and uterus of the mother. It is carried out for various medical reasons; the mother usually recovers quickly, without complications. The procedure is named after Julius Caesar (100–44 BC), who is reputed to have been born this way.

birth control *See* CONTRACEPTION

Black Death (1347–52) Pandemic of PLAGUE, both bubonic and pneumonic, which killed

B

◀ *Black Death* *False-colour TEM of* Yersinia pestis, *the bacterium which causes bubonic plague (the Black Death of the Middle Ages). According to the World Health Organization, the bacterium continues to kill about 3,000 people each year.*

blood clotting Protective mechanism that prevents excessive blood loss after injury. A mesh of tight fibres (of insoluble FIBRIN) coagulates at the site of injury through a complex series of chemical reactions. This mesh traps blood cells to form a clot, which dries to form a scab. This prevents further loss of blood, and also prevents BACTERIA getting into the wound. Normal clotting takes place within five minutes. The clotting mechanism is impaired in some diseases, such as HAEMOPHILIA. *See* p. 67

blood group Any of the types into which blood is classified according to which ANTI-GENS are present on the surface of its red cells. There are four major types: A, B, AB and O. Each group in the ABO system may also contain the rhesus factor (Rh), in which case it is Rh-positive: otherwise it is Rh-negative. Such typing is essential before BLOOD TRANSFUSION, since using blood of the wrong group may produce a dangerous or even fatal reaction. *See* p. 67

blood poisoning (septicaemia) Presence in the blood of BACTERIA or their toxins in sufficient quantity to cause illness. Symptoms include chills and fever, sweating and collapse. It is most often seen in people who are already in some way vulnerable, such as the young or old, the critically ill or injured or those whose immune systems have been suppressed.

blood pressure Force exerted by circulating BLOOD on the walls of blood vessels due to the pumping action of the heart. This is measured using a gauge known as a SPHYGMOMANOMETER. It is greatest when the heart contracts, and lowest when it relaxes. High blood pressure is associated with an increased risk of heart attacks and STROKES. Abnormally low blood pressure is mostly seen in people in SHOCK or following excessive loss of fluid or blood.

about one-third of the population of Europe (200 million people) in six years. The plague reached East Asia in the mid-1330s and West Asia a decade later. It was first carried to Mediterranean ports from the Crimea and spread rapidly throughout Europe, carried by fleas infesting rats. Plague recurred less severely in 1361 and other years, until the 18th century.

blindness Severe impairment or absence of sight. It may be due to heredity, accident, disease, or old age. Worldwide, the most common cause of blindness is TRACHOMA. In developed countries, blindness is most often due to severe DIABETES, GLAUCOMA, CATARACT or degenerative changes associated with ageing.

blood Fluid circulating in the body that transports oxygen and nutrients to all the cells and removes wastes such as carbon dioxide. In a healthy human, it constitutes c.5% of the body's total weight; by volume, it comprises c.5.5 l (9.7 pt). It is composed of a colourless, transparent fluid called PLASMA in which are suspended microscopic ERYTHROCYTES, LEUCOCYTES and PLATELETS. *See* pp. 64–66

blood transfusion Transfer of blood or a component of blood from one body to another to make up for a deficiency. This is possible only if the BLOOD GROUPS of the donor and recipient are compatible. It is often done to counteract life-threatening SHOCK following excessive loss of blood. Donated blood is scrutinized before use for readily transmissible diseases such as HEPATITIS B and ACQUIRED IMMUNE DEFICIENCY SYNDROME (AIDS).

boil (furuncle) Small, pus-filled swelling on the skin, often formed around a hair follicle or sebaceous gland. Most boils are caused by infection from a bacterium (STAPHYLOCOCCUS).

boric acid (boracic acid) Soft, white crystalline solid (H_3BO_3) that occurs naturally in certain volcanic hot springs. It is used as a metallurgical flux, preservative, antiseptic and an insecticide for pests.

botulism Rare, but potentially lethal, form of food poisoning caused by a toxin produced by the bacterium *Clostridium botulinum*. The toxin attacks the nervous system, causing paralysis and cessation of breathing. The most likely source of botulism is imperfectly canned meat. Botulinum toxin (**Botox**) is used medicinally as a treatment for some neuromuscular disorders and in plastic surgery.

bovine spongiform encephalopathy (BSE) In cattle, degeneration of the brain caused by infectious particles or PRIONS, which may be transmitted by feeding infected meat. It is also known as 'mad cow disease'. From 1986 to 2000, more than 4.5 million BSE-infected cattle were slaughtered in the United Kingdom. *See also* CREUTZFELDT-JAKOB DISEASE (CJD)

brain damage Result of any harm done to brain tissue causing the death of nerve cells. It may arise from a number of causes, such as oxygen deprivation, brain or other disease or head injury. The nature and extent of damage varies. Sudden failure of the oxygen supply to the brain may result in widespread (global) damage, whereas a blow to the head may affect only one part of the brain (local damage). Common effects of brain damage include weakness of one or more limbs, impaired balance, memory loss and personality change; epilepsy may develop. While brain cells do not regenerate, there is some hope of improvement following mild to moderate brain damage, especially with skilled rehabilitation. The survivor of major brain injury is likely to remain severely disabled, possibly even permanently unconscious.

breathing Process by which air is taken into and expelled from the lungs for the

▶ *Blood clot Coloured SEM of a blood clot. Red blood cells are seen trapped in a web of white fibrin threads made of an insoluble protein. Small platelets (green) have also become enmeshed. When activated, platelets become spiky (as here), clump together and release chemicals into the blood. These factors cause fibrin threads to form. A white blood cell is also trapped (yellow). A clot that forms inside a blood vessel may lead to a heart attack if it blocks a heart artery. Magnification: ×4,200.*

B

purpose of gas exchange. During inhalation, the intercostal muscles raise the ribs, increasing the volume of the thorax and drawing air into the lungs. During exhalation, the ribs are lowered, and air is forced out through the nose and sometimes also the mouth. *See* pp. 78–79

British Medical Association (BMA) UK professional body founded in 1832: 66% of all doctors in Britain are members. The BMA was set up in order to advance the medical sciences. Since the establishment of the UK NATIONAL HEALTH SERVICE (NHS) in 1948, it has also negotiated pay and conditions for hospital doctors and general practitioners.

bronchitis Inflammation of the bronchial tubes, most often caused by a viral infection such as the common cold or influenza but exacerbated by environmental pollutants. Symptoms include coughing and the production of large quantities of mucus. It can be acute (sudden and short-lived) or chronic (persistent), especially in those who smoke.

BSE *See* BOVINE SPONGIFORM ENCEPHALOPATHY

bubonic plague *See* PLAGUE

bulimia nervosa Eating disorder that takes the form of compulsive eating, then purging by induced vomiting or the use of a LAXATIVE or DIURETIC. Confined mainly to girls and women, the disorder most often results from an underlying psychological problem. An obsession with body image may be reinforced by Western media stereotypes of 'slim as beautiful'. *See also* ANOREXIA NERVOSA

burn Injury caused by exposure to flames, scalding liquids, caustic chemicals, acids, electric current or ionizing radiation. Its severity depends on the extent of skin loss and the depth of tissue damage. A **superficial** burn, involving only the epidermis (the outer later of the skin, without blood vessels), causes redness, swelling and pain: it heals within a few days. A **partial thickness** burn (epidermis and dermis) causes intense pain, with mottling and

blistering of the skin: it takes a couple of weeks to heal. In a **full thickness** burn, involving both the skin and the underlying flesh, there is charring and the damaged flesh looks dry and leathery, although there is no pain because the nerve endings have been destroyed. Such a burn, serious in itself, is associated with life-threatening complications including dehydration and infection. Treatment includes fluid replacement and antibiotics and skin-grafting may be necessary.

bursitis Inflammation of the fluid-filled sac (bursa) surrounding a joint. It is characterized by pain, swelling and restricted movement. Treatment generally includes rest, heat and gentle exercise. 'Housemaid's knee', 'tennis elbow' and bunions are common forms of bursitis.

Caesarean section *See* BIRTH, CAESAREAN

caffeine ($C_8H_{10}N_4O_2$) White, bitter substance that occurs in coffee, tea and other substances, such as cocoa and ilex plants. It acts as a mild, harmless stimulant and DIURETIC, although an excessive dose can cause insomnia and delirium.

cancer Group of diseases featuring the uncontrolled proliferation of cells (TUMOUR formation). Malignant (cancerous) cells spread (metastasize) from their original site to other parts of the body. There are many different cancers. Known causative agents (carcinogens) include tobacco smoke, certain industrial chemicals, asbestos dust and radioactivity. Viruses are implicated in the causation of some cancers. Some people have a genetic tendency towards particular types of cancer. Treatments include surgery, chemotherapy with cell-destroying drugs and radiotherapy (or sometimes a combination of all three). Early diagnosis holds out the best chance of successful treatment.

carbohydrate Organic compound of carbon, hydrogen and oxygen. The simplest carbohydrates are sugars. Glucose and fructose are monosaccharides, naturally occurring sugars; they have the same formula ($C_6H_{12}O_6$) but different structures. One molecule of each combines with the loss of water to make sucrose ($C_{12}H_{22}O_{11}$), a disaccharide. Starch and cellulose are polysaccharides – carbohydrates consisting of hundreds of glucose molecules linked together.

carcinoma Form of CANCER arising from the epithelial cells present in skin and the membranes lining the internal organs. It is a malignant growth that can increase and invade surrounding tissues, giving rise to further metastases (secondary cancers).

There are two main types of carcinoma: basal cell (or rodent ulcer) and squamous cell. Both are related to sunlight exposure. *See also* MELANOMA; SARCOMA

cardiology Branch of medicine that deals with the diagnosis and treatment of the diseases and disorders of the heart and vascular system.

C

castration Removal of the sexual glands (testes or ovaries) from an animal or human. In human beings, removal of the testes has been used as a form of punishment, a way of sexually incapacitating slaves to produce eunuchs (who were often left in charge of harems), a way of artificially creating soprano voices (castrato) and as a method of stopping the spread of cancer. The procedure can also make animals tamer.

catabolism *See* METABOLISM

cataract Opacity in the lens of an eye, causing blurring of vision. Most cases are due to degenerative changes in old age but it can also be congenital, the result of damage to

► *Cancer can spread in two ways. First, by direct growth into adjacent tissues, called 'direct extension' (A), when cancer cells penetrate into bone, soft connective tissue and the walls of veins and lymphatic vessels. Second. by 'metastasis' (B), when a cancer cell separates from its tumour and is transported to another part of the body. After the tumour has grown to some size, cancer cells or small groups of cells enter a blood or lymph vessel through the vessel wall (1). They travel through the vessel until they hit a barrier, such as a lymph node, where additional tumours may develop, before releasing more cells* which may develop on other lymph nodes. Such cancers, usually carcinomas, may also invade the bloodstream and establish more distant secondary growths. Another type of cancer, sarcomas, tend to spread via venous blood vessels establishing tumours in the lungs, gastrointestinal tract or genito-urinary tract (2). In abdominal cancers, metastases may also arise through travel across body cavities, such as the peritoneal, oral or pleural cavities (3).

C

◄ *Cerebral haemorrhage* Computer artwork of the blood vessels in the human head, showing an intracerebral brain haemorrhage which may lead to a cerebrovascular accident, or stroke. The large orange area at top left is a blood-filled area, or brain haemorrhage. This can be caused by a head injury or by the spontaneous rupture of a blood vessel. The carotid arteries carry blood from the body's main artery, the aorta (seen at bottom centre) to the head. Stroke is a major cause of death in developed countries. If patients survive, damage to the brain can cause varied symptoms, such as weakness or paralysis. Brain haemorrhages divide into four main categories – extradural, subdural, subarachnoid and intracerebral – according to the site of the bleeding.

the lens or a metabolic disorder such as diabetes. Treatment is by removal of the cataract and implantation of an artificial lens.

cephalosporin Class of ANTIBIOTIC drugs derived from fungi of the genus *Cephalosporium*. Similar to PENICILLIN, they are effective against a wide spectrum of BACTERIA, including some which have become resistant to penicillin.

cerebral haemorrhage Form of STROKE in which there is bleeding from a blood vessel in the brain into the surrounding tissue. It is usually caused by ARTERIOSCLEROSIS and high blood pressure. Symptoms may vary from temporary numbness and weakness down one side of the body to deep coma. A major haemorrhage may be fatal. There is a high risk of repeated strokes.

cerebral hemispheres Lateral halves of the cerebrum, the largest parts of the brain and the sites of higher thought. Due to the crossing over of nerve fibres from one cerebral hemisphere to the other, the right side controls most of the movements and sensation on the left side of the body, and vice-versa. Damage to cerebral hemispheres can produce personality changes.

cerebral palsy Disorder mainly of movement and co-ordination caused by damage to the brain during or soon after birth. It may feature muscular spasm and weakness, lack of co-ordination, and impaired movement or paralysis and deformities of the limbs. Intelligence is not necessarily affected. The condition may result from a number of causes, such as faulty development, oxygen deprivation, birth injury, haemorrhage or infection.

cerebrospinal fluid Clear liquid that cushions the brain and spinal cord, giving some protection against shock. It is found between the two innermost meninges (membranes) in the four ventricles of the brain and in the central canal of the spinal cord. A small quantity of the fluid can be withdrawn by lumbar puncture to aid diagnosis of some brain diseases.

cervical smear (pap test) Test for CANCER of the cervix, established by George Papanikolaou. In this diagnostic procedure, a small sample of tissue is removed from the cervix and examined under a microscope for the presence of abnormal, pre-cancerous cells. Treatment in the early stages of cervical cancer can prevent the disease from developing.

chemotherapy Treatment of a disease (usually cancer) by a combination of chemical substances, or drugs, that kill or impair disease-producing organisms in the body. Specific drug treatment was introduced in the early 1900s by Paul Ehrlich.

chickenpox (varicella) Infectious disease of childhood caused by a virus of the HERPES group. After an incubation period of two to three weeks, a fever develops and red spots (which later develop into blisters) appear on the trunk, face and limbs. Recovery is usual within a week, although the possibility of contagion remains until the last scab has been shed.

childbirth See LABOUR

chiropractic Non-orthodox medical practice based on the theory that the nervous system integrates all of the body's functions, including defence against disease. Chiropractors aim to remove nerve interference by manipulations of the affected musculo-skeletal parts, particularly in the spinal region.

chlamydia Small, simple BACTERIA that live as PARASITES in animals and cause disease.

One strain, *C. trachomatis*, causes TRACHOMA and is also a major cause of pelvic inflammatory disease (PID) in women. *C. psittaci* causes PSITTACOSIS. Chlamydial infection is the most common SEXUALLY TRANSMITTED DISEASE (STD) in many developed countries.

chloroform (trichloromethane) Colourless, volatile, sweet-smelling liquid ($CHCl_3$) prepared by the chlorination of methane. Formerly a major anaesthetic, it is used in the manufacture of fluorocarbons, in cough medicines, for insect bites and as a solvent. Properties: r.d. 1.48; m.p. –63.5°C (–82.3°F); b.p. 61.2°C (142.2°F).

cholera Infectious disease caused by the bacterium *Vibrio cholerae*, transmitted in contaminated water. Cholera, prevalent in many tropical regions, produces almost continuous, watery DIARRHOEA often accompanied by vomiting and muscle cramps, and leads to severe dehydration. Untreated it can be fatal, but proper treatment, including fluid replacement and antibiotics, result in a high recovery rate. There is a vaccine.

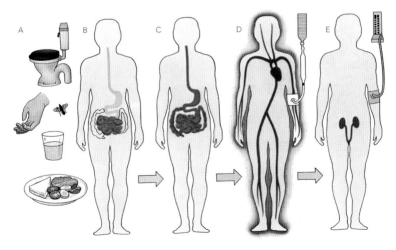

▲ *Cholera is one of the many diseases that spread because of poor hygiene. Human faeces containing cholera germs contaminate food and water (A). The victim ingests them and they incubate in his small intestine (B). They then produce severe, often fatal diarrhoea (C). The patient may survive if this gross dehydration can be corrected with intravenous fluid (D). If such therapy is undertaken promptly (and if no kidney damage has occurred) then full recovery should take place (E).*

cholesterol White, fatty STEROID, occurring in large concentrations in the brain, spinal cord and liver. It is synthesized in the liver, intestines and skin and is an intermediate in the synthesis of vitamin D and many hormones. GALLSTONES are composed mainly of cholesterol. Meat-rich diets may produce high cholesterol in blood vessels, and can lead to atherosclerosis. *See also* ARTERIOSCLEROSIS

chromosome Structure carrying genetic information, found only in the cell nucleus of eukaryotes. Thread-like and composed of DNA, chromosomes carry a specific set of genes. Each species usually has a characteristic number of chromosomes: these occur in pairs, members of which carry identical genes, so that most cells are diploid. Gametes carry a haploid number of chromosomes.

circadian rhythm Internal 'clock' mechanism found in most organisms. It normally corresponds with the 24-hour day, relating most obviously to waking and sleeping cycles, but is also involved in other cyclic variations, such as body temperature, hormone levels, metabolism and mental performance.

circumcision Operation of removing part or the whole of the foreskin of the penis or of removing the clitoris. Male circumcision is ritual in some groups, notably Jews and Muslims, and is said to have sanitary benefits: Female circumcision is intended to reduce sexual pleasure and has no medical benefit.

cirrhosis Degenerative disease in which there is excessive growth of fibrous tissue in an organ, most often the liver, causing inflammation and scarring. Cirrhosis of the liver may be caused by viral hepatitis, prolonged obstruction of the common bile duct, chronic abuse of alcohol or other drugs, blood disorder, heart failure or malnutrition.

cleft palate Congenital deformity in which there is an opening in the roof of the mouth, causing direct communication between the nasal and mouth cavities. It is often associated with HARELIP and makes normal speech difficult. Usual treatment includes surgical correction, followed by special dental care and speech therapy if necessary.

clone Set of organisms obtained from a single original parent either by asexual reproduction or by artificial selection. Clones are genetically identical and may arise naturally from parthenogenesis in animals. Cloning is often used in plant propagation (including tissue culture) to produce new plants from parents with desirable qualities such as high yield. In 1996 scientists in Scotland produced a sheep embryo from a single cell of an adult sheep using nuclear-transfer technology (transfer of a cell nucleus). *See also* GENETIC ENGINEERING

coca Shrub native to Colombia and Peru which contains the alkaloid drug COCAINE. Native Americans chew the leaves for pleasure, to quell hunger and to stimulate the nervous system. The plant has

◄ **Coca** *Native to regions of South America, the leaves of the coca tree (Erythroxylon coca) have been used for centuries as medicine and to relieve hunger. The leaves are harvested and used in the illegal manufacture of cocaine. The narcotic principle is the alkaloid cocaine, of which the leaves contain about 1%.*

yellow-white flowers growing in clusters, and red berries. Height of shrub: c.2.4 m (8 ft). Family Erythroxylaceae; species *Erythroxylon coca*.

cocaine White, crystalline alkaloid extracted from the leaves of the COCA plant. Once used as a local anaesthetic, it is now primarily an illegal narcotic with stimulant and hallucinatory effects. It is psychologically habit-forming and the body does not develop tolerance. Habitual use of cocaine results in physical and nervous deterioration and subsequent withdrawal results in severe depression. *See also* CRACK

coccus Small spherical or spheroid bacterium. Average diameter: 0.0005–0.0012 mm (0.00002–0.00004 in). Some, such as *Streptococcus* and *Staphylococcus*, are common causes of infection.

codeine White, crystalline alkaloid extracted from OPIUM by the methylation of MORPHINE, with the properties of weak morphine. It is used in medicine as an analgesic to treat mild to moderate pain, as a cough suppressant and to treat diarrhoea.

cold, common Minor disease of the upper respiratory tract caused by viral infection. Symptoms include inflammation of the nose, headache, sore throat and a cough. A cold usually disappears within a few days. Fever-reducing and pain-relieving drugs, as well as decongestants, may relieve symptoms. Rest is recommended for heavy colds. Antibiotics may be prescribed where a bacterial infection is also present.

colic Severe pain in the abdomen, usually becoming intense, subsiding and then recurring. Intestinal colic may be associated with obstruction of the intestine or constipation.

colitis Inflammation of the lining of the colon, or large intestine, that produces bowel changes, usually diarrhoea and cramp-like pains. In severe chronic ulcerative colitis, the colon lining ulcerates and bleeds.

collagen Protein substance that is the main constituent of bones, tendons, cartilage, connective tissue and skin. It is made up of inelastic fibres.

colostomy Operation to bring the colon out through the wall of the abdomen in order to bypass the lower section of the bowel. An artificial opening is created so that faecal matter is passed into a bag, worn outside the body. The site of the colostomy varies according to the disease's location.

colour blindness General term for various disorders of colour vision. The most common involves red-green vision, a hereditary defect almost exclusively affecting males. Total colour blindness (achromatic vision), an inherited disorder in which the person sees only black, white and grey, is very rare. *See* p. 53

coma State of unconsciousness brought about by head injury, brain disease, drugs or lack of blood supply to the brain.

congenital disorder Abnormal condition present from birth caused by faulty development, infection or the mother's exposure to drugs or other toxic substances during pregnancy. SPINA BIFIDA is such a condition.

contact lens Lens worn on the cornea of the eye to aid defective vision. Invented in 1887, lenses were initially made of glass. Modern contact lenses, developed (1948) by Kevin Tuohy, are made of plastic. **Hard** (corneal) lenses cover the pupil and part of the cornea. They are usually gas-permeable (allowing oxygen to reach the cornea). **Soft** (hydrophilic) lenses cover the whole cornea and are hydrated in saline solution.

contraception (birth control) Use of devices or techniques to prevent PREGNANCY. The PILL is a hormone preparation that prevents the release of an egg (ovum) and thickens the cervical mucus. Barrier methods include the male and female condom and the diaphragm. The male **condom** is a latex sheath that covers the penis and

◄ *Contraception Methods include a condom or sheath (A) over the penis preventing sperm from entering the vagina, or a cap (B) over the cervix preventing sperm from entering the uterus. Spermicidal foams and jellies (C) placed in the vagina will kill sperm at this point. More permanent forms of contraception are operations tying off the vas deferens (vasectomy, D) or the oviduct (tubar ligation, E). Ovulation by the ovary (F) may be prevented by the oral contraceptive pill.*

collects the ejaculated semen while the female condom lines the inside of the vagina, preventing any sperm entering the womb. The use of condoms is widely advocated because they protect against some SEXUALLY TRANSMITTED DISEASES (STDs), including ACQUIRED IMMUNE DEFICIENCY SYNDROME (AIDS). Devices, such as the diaphragm or cap, cover the cervix thus preventing sperm entering the womb. Less effective is the 'rhythm method', which involves the avoidance of sex on days when conception is most likely (when the woman is ovulating). It is not a reliable method as ovulation cannot always be predicted accurately. Emergency contraception, known as the 'morning-after pill', can be taken up to 72 hours after unprotected sexual intercourse: it prevents the fertilized ovum embedding itself in the womb. It is not suitable to be used regularly.

convulsion Intense, involuntary contraction of the muscles, sometimes accompanied by loss of consciousness. A seizure may indicate EPILEPSY although there are other causes, including intoxication, brain abscess or HYPOGLYCAEMIA.

coronary artery disease Disease of the coronary blood vessels, particularly the aorta and arteries supplying blood to the heart. *See also* ANGINA; ARTERIOSCLEROSIS

coronary heart disease ARTERIOSCLEROSIS of the coronary arteries. It is the most common cause of death in the West. Atheriosclerosis can lead to the formation of a blood clot in one or other of the coronary arteries supplying the heart (**coronary thrombosis**). The patient experiences sudden pain in the chest (ANGINA) and the result may be a HEART ATTACK (**myocardial infarction**), when the flow of blood to the heart is stopped. Smokers are more likely to die suddenly from atheriosclerosis. Evidence suggests that a high intake of polyunsaturated fats can protect against coronary heart disease.

cortisone Hormone produced by the cortex of the adrenal glands (on top of the kidneys) and essential for carbohydrate, protein and fat METABOLISM, kidney function and disease resistance. Synthetic cortisone is used to treat adrenal insufficiency, rheumatoid arthritis and other inflammatory diseases and rheumatic fever. *See also* p. 57

cot death *See* SUDDEN INFANT DEATH SYNDROME (SIDS)

crack Street DRUG that is a COCAINE derivative. It is supplied in the form of hard, crystalline lumps, which are heated to produce smoke inhaled for its stimulant effects. It imposes considerable strain on the heart and blood vessels and may result in heart failure or a stroke. Psychotic episodes may also occur.

Creutzfeldt-Jakob disease (CJD) Rare, degenerative brain disease that causes physical deterioration and dementia, usually leading to death within a year of onset. Caused by an abnormal protein (a prion), it is related to scrapie in sheep and 'mad cow disease', or BOVINE SPONGIFORM ENCEPHALOPATHY (BSE). Typically it affects older people, but in 1996 scientists found a new variant form of CJD (nvCJD) in younger victims. In 1997 research confirmed that the agent responsible for this variant was identical to that of BSE, confirming the link between CJD and the consumption of infected beef. There is currently no known cure.

croup Respiratory disorder of children caused by inflammation of the larynx (voice box) and airways. It is triggered by viral infection. Symptoms are a cough, difficulty in breathing and fever.

CT scan (computed tomography) X-ray technique for displaying images of cross-sections through the human body. X-ray sources and detectors slowly move around the patient's body on opposite sides, producing a changing 'view' of an organ. The data from the detectors is processed through a computer to display only the details relating to a specific 'slice' through the body.

curare Poisonous resinous extract obtained from various tropical South American plants of the genera *Chondodendron* and *Strychnos*. Most of its active elements are alkaloids. It is used as a muscle relaxant in abdominal surgery and setting fractures.

cystic fibrosis Hereditary glandular disease in which the body produces abnormally thick mucus that obstructs the breathing passages, causing chronic lung disease. There is a deficiency of pancreatic

▶ *Creutzfeldt-Jakob disease (CJD)* Coloured Magnetic Resonance Imaging (MRI) scan of the brain of a 17-year-old male suffering from Creutzfeldt-Jakob disease (CJD: new variant) in 1997. The patient died. The front of the head is at top. In this axial 'slice' through the brain, the folded cerebrum is seen forming two hemispheres. At lower centre are two red areas of the thalamus diseased with CJD. It is detected as a 'bilateral signal abnormality' on MRI. CJD destroys nerve cells and causes brain tissue to become spongy. Symptoms include dementia, muscle contractions and death. There is concern that eating beef from 'mad cows' may cause CJD.

131

► **Cystic fibrosis** *Coloured SEM of mucus in a bronchus of the lung of a patient suffering cystic fibrosis. A large clump of mucus is at centre (red). The bronchial airways are lined with hair-like cilia (green, yellow). At top, rounded goblet cells (blue) secrete the mucus that catches inhaled particles. People with cystic fibrosis suffer chronic infection of and mucus production in the lungs.*

C

enzymes, an abnormally high salt concentration in the sweat and a general failure to gain weight. The disease is treated with antibiotics, pancreatic enzymes and a high-protein diet. Sufferers must undergo vigorous physiotherapy to keep the chest as clear as possible.

cystitis Inflammation of the urinary bladder, usually caused by bacterial infection. It is more common in women. Symptoms include frequent and painful urination, low back pain and slight fever.

deafness Partial or total hearing loss. **Conductive** deafness, faulty transmission of sound to the sensory organs, is usually due to infection or inherited abnormalities of the middle ear. **Perceptive** deafness may be hereditary or due to injury or disease of the cochlea in the ear, auditory

nerve or hearing centres in the brain. Treatment of deafness ranges from removal of impacted wax to delicate microsurgery. Hearing aids, sign language and lip-reading are some of the different techniques which help deaf people to communicate. *See pp. 54–5*

death Cessation of life. In medicine, death has traditionally been pronounced on cessation of the heartbeat. However, modern resuscitation and life-support techniques have enabled the revival of patients whose hearts have stopped. In a tiny minority of cases, while breathing and heartbeat can be maintained artificially, the potential for life is extinct. In this context, death may be pronounced when it is clear that the brain no longer controls vital functions. The issue is highly controversial.

decompression sickness *See* BENDS

dehydration Removal or loss of water from a substance or tissue. Water molecules can be removed by heat, catalysts or a dehydrating agent such as concentrated sulphuric acid. Dehydration is used in food preservation. In medicine, excessive water loss is often a symptom or result of disease or injury.

delirium State of confusion in which a person becomes agitated and incoherent and loses touch with reality. It is often associated with delusions or HALLUCINATIONS.

Delusion may be seen in various disorders, brain disease, fever and drug or alcohol intoxication.

dementia Deterioration of personality and intellect that can result from disease of, or damage to, the brain. It is characterized by memory loss, impaired mental processes, personality change, confusion, lack of inhibition and deterioration in personal hygiene. Dementia can occur at any age, although it is more common in the elderly. *See also* ALZHEIMER'S DISEASE

dengue Infectious virus disease transmitted by the *Aedes aegypti* mosquito. Occurring in the tropics and some temperate areas, it produces fever, headache and fatigue, followed by severe joint pains, aching muscles, swollen glands and a rash.

dentistry Profession concerned with the care and treatment of the mouth, particularly the teeth and their supporting

tissues. As well as general practice, dentistry includes specialities such as oral surgery, periodontics and orthodontics.

dermatitis Inflammation of the skin. In acute form, it produces itching and blisters. In chronic form, it causes thickening, scaling and darkening of the skin. *See also* ECZEMA

dermatology Branch of medicine that deals with the diagnosis and treatment of skin diseases.

diabetes Disease characterized by lack of INSULIN needed for sugar METABOLISM. This leads to HYPERGLYCAEMIA and an excess of sugar in the blood. Symptoms include abnormal thirst, overproduction of urine, and weight loss. In addition, degenerative changes occur in blood vessels. Untreated, the condition progresses to diabetic coma and death. There are two forms of the disease. **Type**

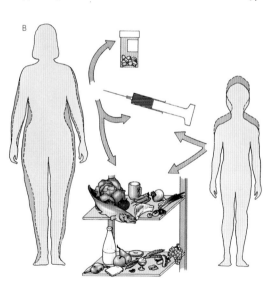

▲ *Diabetes mellitus (A) may cause drowsiness and coma (1), impaired vision (2), dry mouth (3), overbreathing (4), cardiac failure (5), high blood sugar levels (6), fatty liver (7),* kidney and bladder infections (8), itchy skin and delayed healing (9) and weight loss (10). Treatment (B) for juveniles includes a varied low-fat diet, usually with insulin injections. Adults also need a low-fat diet and weight loss, but drugs may help to control the disease. If not, then insulin may be administered.

1 usually begins in childhood and is an autoimmune disease. Those affected owe their survival to insulin injections. **Type 2** diabetes mostly begins in middle-age: there is some insulin output but not enough for the body's needs. The disease can be managed with dietary restrictions, tablets to lower blood sugar levels and insulin injections. Susceptibility to *diabetes mellitus* is inherited and is more common in males.

dialysis Process for separating particles from a solution by virtue of differing rates of diffusion through a semipermeable membrane. In an artificial kidney, unwanted molecules of waste products are separated out to purify the blood. Electrodialysis employs a direct electric current to accelerate the process, which is especially useful for isolating proteins.

diarrhoea Frequent elimination of loose, watery stools, often accompanied by cramps and stomach pains. It arises from various causes, such as infection, intestinal irritants or food allergy. Mild attacks can be treated by replacement fluids.

diet Range of food and drink consumed by an animal. The human diet falls into five main groups of necessary nutrients: PROTEIN, CARBOHYDRATE, FAT, VITAMIN and MINERAL. An adult's daily requirement is about 1 g of protein for each kg of body weight. Beans, fish, eggs, milk and meat are important protein sources. Carbohydrates (stored as glycogen) and fat are the chief sources of energy and are found in cereals, root vegetables and sugars. Carbohydrates make up the bulk of most diets. Fats are a concentrated source of energy and aid the absorption of fat-soluble vitamins (vitamins A, D, E and K). Water and minerals, such as iron, calcium, potassium and sodium, are also essential.

diphtheria Acute infectious disease characterized by the formation of a membrane in the throat which can cause asphyxiation: there is also release of a toxin which can damage the nerves and heart. Caused by a bacterium, *Corynebacterium diphtheri-*

ae, which often enters through the upper respiratory tract, it is treated with antitoxin and antibiotics.

diploid Cell that has its CHROMOSOMES in pairs. Diploids are found in almost all animal cells, except GAMETES which are HAPLOID. In diploids, the chromosomes of each pair carry the same genes.

disease Any departure from health, with impaired functioning of the body. Disease may be **acute** with severe symptoms for a short time; **chronic**, and lasting a long time, or **recurrent** and returning periodically. There are many types and causes of disease: infectious (caused by harmful BACTERIA or viruses), hereditary and metabolic, in growth and development, affecting the immune system, neoplastic (TUMOUR-producing), caused by nutritional deficiency, of the endocrine system or caused by environmental agents, such as lead poisoning. Treatment depends on the cause and course of the disease. It may be **symptomatic** (relieving symptoms, but not necessarily combating a cause) or **specific** (attempting to cure an underlying cause). Disease prevention includes eradication of harmful organisms, VACCINES, public health measures and routine medical checks.

diuretic Drug used to increase the output of urine. It is used to treat raised blood pressure and OEDEMA.

DNA (deoxyribonucleic acid) Molecule found in all cells, and in some VIRUSES, which is responsible for storing the genetic instructions. It consists of two long chains of alternating sugar molecules and phosphate groups linked by nitrogenous bases. The whole molecule is shaped like a twisted rope ladder, with the nitrogenous bases forming the rungs. The sugar is deoxyribose and the four bases are adenine, cytosine, guanine and thymine. A base and its associated sugar are known as a **nucleotide**. The whole chain is a polynucleotide chain. Genetic information is stored in terms of the sequence of bases: three bases code for one specific amino acid and a series of them constitutes a gene. In eukaryote

D

cells, DNA is stored in chromosomes inside the nucleus. Loops of DNA also occur inside chloroplasts and mitochondria. *See also* RNA

dopamine Chemical normally found in the corpus striatum region of the human brain. Insufficient levels are associated with PARKINSON'S DISEASE. Dopamine is a NEUROTRANSMITTER and a precursor in the production of ADRENALINE and NORADRENALINE.

Down's syndrome Human condition caused by a chromosomal abnormality. It gives rise to varying degrees of mental retardation, decreased life expectancy and perhaps physical problems such as heart and respiratory disorders. The syndrome was first described by a British physician, J L H Down. It is caused by the presence of an extra copy of chromosome 21 and is detected by counting chromosomes in the cells of the fetus during pre-natal testing. There is evidence that the risk of having a Down's child increases with maternal age. It was originally called 'Mongolism' by Down, but this term is now obsolete. *See also* Genes and Inheritance, pp. 110–111

dream Mental activity associated with the rapid-eye-movement (REM) period of sleep. It is usually a train of thoughts,

scenes and desires expressed in visual images and symbols. On average, a person dreams for a total of 1.5–2 hours in 8 hours of sleep. Dream content is often connected with body changes. For centuries, dreams have been regarded as a source of prophecy or visionary insight. In psychoanalysis, patients' dreams are often examined to reveal their latent content.

drug In medicine, any substance used to diagnose, prevent or treat disease or aid recovery from injury. Although many drugs are still obtained from natural sources, scientists are continually developing synthetic drugs which work on target cells or microorganisms. Such drugs include ANTIBIOTICS. Some drugs interfere in physiological processes, such as anticoagulants which render the blood less prone to clotting. Drugs also may be given to make good some deficiency, such as hormone preparations which compensate for an underactive gland.

drug addiction Psychological or physical dependence on a DRUG. **Physical** addiction is often manifested by symptoms of withdrawal. Long-term drug use often produces tolerance. Physical addiction has only been medically proven for NARCOTICS (such as HEROIN), depressants (such

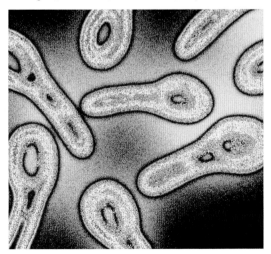

▶ *Diphtheria Coloured TEM of Corynebacterium diphtheriae, the bacterium that causes diphtheria. The bacteria are club-shaped, gram-positive, non-motile rods. They have a spiral nuclear region (red and orange in centre of bacteria) contained within cytoplasm (white speckled). Surrounding each cell is a mucus cell wall (red outlines). Diphtheria is caused by a potent exotoxin released from the bacterium. Symptoms include sore throat, fever and breathing difficulties. Magnification: x30,000.*

as BARBITURATES or alcohol) and some STIM-ULANTS (such as NICOTINE). Other drugs, such as hallucinogens or hashish, are not thought to be physically addictive, but can produce PSYCHOSIS or paranoia. Two of the most common addictions are alcohol and nicotine, since these are easily available. Unlike narcotics, alcohol is physically harmful, especially to the brain and liver, and cigarette smoking annually accounts for more than 100,000 premature deaths in the United Kingdom alone. In comparison, addiction to 'hard' drugs (such as HEROIN or COCAINE) is not common, but drug-related crime makes up a significant percentage of crime statistics in many countries.

dysentery Infectious disease characterized by DIARRHOEA, bleeding and abdominal cramps. It spreads in contaminated food and water, especially in the tropics. There are two types: **bacillary** dysentery, caused by BACTERIA of the genus *Shigella*, and **amoebic** dysentery, caused by a type of protist (unicellular organism). Both forms are treated with antibacterials and fluid replacement.

dyspepsia (indigestion) Pain or discomfort in the stomach or abdomen arising from digestive upset.

ebola Virus that causes haemorrhagic fever. Thought to have been long present in animals, the ebola virus was first identified in humans during an outbreak in Congo in 1976. It is acquired through contact with contaminated body fluids. Death rates can be as high as 90%.

ecstasy (MDMA) (3,4–methylenedioxy-methylamphetamine) AMPHETAMINE-based drug, which raises body temperature and blood pressure by inducing the release of adrenaline and targeting the neurotransmitter serotonin. Users experience short-term feelings of euphoria, rushes of energy and increased tactility. Withdrawal can involve bouts of depression and INSOMNIA.

◀ *Ectopic pregnancy* An ectopic or extrauterine pregnancy occurs when the egg, released from the ovary (*1*) and fertilized by the sperm (*2*) in the fallopian tube (*3*), fails to pass down into the uterus (*4*) where it would normally implant in the wall of the womb (*5*). If the zygote implants in the wall of the fallopian tube (*6*), there is not enough space or the blood supply to nurture a fetus to full term and the pregnancy usually aborts spontaneously. If not, surgery is necessary to remove the fetus and save the mother.

► *Embolism* *Illustration of a venous embolism (obstruction) caused by a thrombus (clot) lodged in a vein. The clot (red) is seen resting in the cusp of a valve that prevents backflow of blood in the vein. The clot is in a region of disturbed blood flow, notably near the valve. Thrombosis (clot formation) may be caused by disturbed blood flow, together with some condition that increases the natural tendency of the blood to clot.*

E

Since the 1980s the consumption of ecstasy in tablet form has been widespread in club cultures in Europe and North America. Today, it is estimated that there are up to 500,000 weekly users in the United Kingdom alone. Deaths have resulted from use of the drug – mostly due to dehydration.

ECT Abbreviation of ELECTROCONVULSIVE THERAPY

ectopic Occurrence of a pregnancy outside the uterus, such as in the fallopian tube. The embryo cannot develop normally, and spontaneous ABORTION (miscarriage) often occurs. If not, urgent surgery is necessary to save the mother from serious haemorrhage. *See also* p. 104–105

eczema Inflammatory condition of the skin, a form of DERMATITIS characterized by dryness, itching, rashes and blister formation. It can be caused by contact with a substance, such as a detergent to which the skin has been sensitized, or a general ALLERGY. Treatment is usually with a corticosteroid ointment.

electrocardiogram (ECG) Recording of the electrical activity of the heart, traced on a moving strip of paper by an electrocardiograph. It is used to diagnose heart disease.

electroconvulsive therapy (ECT) Treatment of mental disturbance by means of an electric current passed via electrodes to one or both sides of the brain to induce convulsions. Given under anaesthesia, it is recommended mainly for depression that has failed to respond to other treatments. It can produce unpleasant side-effects, such as confu-

sion, memory loss and headache. It is a highly controversial form of therapy.

electroencephalogram (EEG) Recording of electrical activity of the brain. Electrodes are attached to the scalp to pick up the tiny oscillating currents produced by brain activity. It is used mainly in the diagnosis and monitoring of EPILEPSY.

elephantiasis Condition in which there is gross swelling of the tissues due to blockage of lymph vessels. It is usually caused by parasitic worms, as in FILARIASIS.

embolism Blocking of a blood vessel by an obstruction called an embolus, usually a blood clot, air bubble or particle of fat. The effects depend on where the embolus lodges; a cerebral embolism causes a STROKE. Treatment is with anticoagulants or surgery. *See also* ARTERIOSCLEROSIS

emphysema Accumulation of air in tissues, usually occurring in the lungs (pulmonary emphysema). Pulmonary emphysema, characterized by marked breathlessness, is the

E

result of damage to and enlargement of the alveoli (tiny air sacs in the lungs). This type of emphysema is associated with chronic bronchitis and smoking.

encephalitis Inflammation of the brain, usually associated with a viral infection: often there is an associated MENINGITIS. Symptoms include fever, headache, lassitude and intolerance of light. In severe cases there may be sensory and behavioural disturbances, paralysis, convulsions and even coma. Tests on CEREBROSPINAL FLUID provide a diagnosis of encephalitis.

endometriosis Gynaecological disorder in which tissue similar to the ENDOMETRIUM is found in other parts of the pelvic cavity. It is treated with analgesics, hormone preparations or surgery.

endometrium Mucous membrane, well supplied with blood vessels, that lines the uterus. The endometrium sheds each month as part of the MENSTRUAL CYCLE. *See also* pp. 100–101

endorphin (endogenous morphine) Naturally occurring peptide NEUROTRANSMITTER found in the pituitary gland that has similar pain-relieving effects to MORPHINE and other derivatives of OPIUM. Endorphins block the sensation of pain by binding to pain-receptor sites. Two endorphins (**enkephalins**) occur in the brain, spinal cord and gut. *See also* ANALGESIC

endoscope Instrument used to examine the interior of the body. Early types of endoscope, such as the opthalmoscope, were developed in the 19th century. Fibre optics has revolutionized the design of endoscopes. The modern endoscope is a flexible, fibreglass instrument that can be swallowed by a patient or introduced through a tiny incision in the body. Most endoscopy is for diagnostic purposes, but endoscopes are also used in biopsy and MINIMAL ACCESS SURGERY.

enzyme (Gk. zymosis, 'fermentation') Protein that functions as a catalyst in biochemical reactions. They remain chemically unaltered in these reactions and so

are effective in tiny quantities. Chemical reactions can occur several thousand or million times faster with enzymes than without. They operate within a narrow temperature range, usually 30°C to 40°C (86°F to 104°F) and have optimal pH ranges. Many enzymes have to be bound to non-protein molecules to function. These molecules include trace elements (such as metals) and co-enzymes (such as vitamins).

epidemic Outbreak of an infectious disease rapidly spreading to many people. The study of epidemics, which includes causes, patterns of contagion and methods of containment, is known as **epidemiology**. An epidemic sweeping across many countries, such as the BLACK DEATH, is termed a pandemic.

epilepsy Disorder characterized by abnormal electrical discharges in the brain which provoke seizures. It is seen both in generalized forms, involving the whole of the cerebral cortex (largest section of the brain), or in partial (focal) attacks arising in one small part of the brain. Attacks are often presaged by warning symptoms, the 'aura'. Seizure types vary from the momentary loss of awareness seen in *petit mal* attacks ('absences') to the major convulsions of *grand mal* epilepsy. Attacks may be triggered by a number of factors, including sleep deprivation, flashing lights or excessive noise. All forms of epilepsy are controlled with anti-convulsant drugs.

erythrocyte Red blood cell, usually disc-shaped and without a nucleus. It contains HAEMOGLOBIN, which combines with oxygen and gives blood its red colour. Normal human blood contains an average of 5 million such cells per cu mm (0.0003 fl oz) of blood.

ethanol (ethyl alcohol C_2H_5OH) Colourless, intoxicating compound with distinctive odour found in alcoholic drinks including wine and beer. Acts as a central nervous system depressant, producing euphoria in small doses and slowed cognition, stupefaction and coma in higher doses.

excretion Elimination of materials from the body that have been involved in METABOLISM. Such waste materials, particularly nitrogenous wastes, would be toxic if allowed to accumulate. In mammals, these wastes excrete mainly as URINE and to some extent by sweating. Carbon dioxide excretes through the lungs during breathing. Defecation is not excretion, as faeces consist mostly of material that has never been part of the body. *See* pp. 82–93

fainting (syncope) Temporary loss of consciousness accompanied by general weakness of the muscles. A faint may be preceded by giddiness, nausea and sweating. Its causes include insufficient flow of blood to the brain and SHOCK.

family planning Alternative term for CONTRACEPTION

famine Extreme prolonged shortage of food, produced by both natural and manmade causes. If it persists, famine results in widespread starvation and death. Famine is often associated with drought or alterations in weather patterns, which leads to crop failure and the destruction of livestock. However, warfare and complex political situations resulting in the mismanagement of food resources are equally likely causes.

fertility drugs Drugs taken to increase a woman's chances of conception and pregnancy. One cause of female sterility is insufficient secretion of pituitary hormones: this can be treated with human chorionic gonadotropin (HCG) or clomiphene citrate, although use of the latter can result in multiple births. In cases where fertilization occurs, but where the uterine lining is unable to support the fetus, the hormone PROGESTERONE may be used. Infertility cannot always be corrected with drugs.

fever Elevation of the body temperature above normal, that is 37°C (98.6°F). It is mostly caused by bacterial or viral infection and can accompany virtually any infectious disease.

fibrin Insoluble, fibrous protein that is essential to BLOOD CLOTTING. Developed in the blood from a soluble protein, fibrinogen, fibrin is laid down at the site of a wound in the form of a mesh, which then dries and hardens so the bleeding stops.

F

▶ *Filariasis Coloured light micrograph (LM) of a Loa loa worm on a human blood smear. The worm can be seen amongst the red blood cells (coloured grey). The Loa loa worm is a parasitic nematode that lives under human skin, causing a form of filariasis called loiasis. The worms are spread by bloodsucking Chrysops flies in tropical Africa, and reach 3–7 cm (1.2–3 in) when mature. Magnification unknown.*

F

filariasis Group of tropical diseases caused by infection with a nematode worm, *filaria*. The parasites, which are transmitted by insects, infiltrate the lymph glands, causing swelling and impaired drainage. Drug treatment reduces the symptoms. *See picture*, p. 139

first aid Action taken by anyone encountering sudden illness or injury in order to save life, mitigate harm or assist subsequent treatment. Properly administered first aid can save lives and improve the extent and speed of recovery. If the victim appears to have a broken bone or internal injuries, they should not be moved. If the victim is unconscious, their head should be turned to one side to prevent choking. Check that the victim has an open airway – if not, they may have respiratory failure (asphyxia). **Asphyxia** may be caused by the obstruction of air passages, in which case the HEIMLICH MANOEUVRE is recommended. For asphyxia caused by fumes or gas, such as carbon monoxide, the victim should be moved to a clear atmosphere before administering artificial respiration. The best method of **artifical respiration** is mouth-to-mouth resuscitation. Place the victim on their back, put one hand under the victim's chin and the other on the forehead. Tilt the victim's head back by lifting with the hand under the chin and pressing down on the forehead. If the victim is a child, take a breath, place your mouth over both the nose and mouth and blow gently. Remove your mouth and listen for air entering the child's lungs. Take a breath and repeat every three seconds until the child begins to breathe. If the victim is an adult, pinch the nostrils shut, take a deep breath, cover the mouth tightly and breathe hard. Repeat this procedure every five seconds. If the victim has swallowed a poisonous substance, identify the **poison** and then call the emergency services. They may recommend inducing vomiting with syrup of ipecac. In the case of animal **bites and stings**, the wound should be cleaned with soap and water before applying antiseptic and a bandage. For poisonous SNAKEBITE, the wound should be cooled with ice to slow down the absorption of poison. A few snakebites require anti-venoms. In order to stop the victim **bleeding** severely, apply direct pressure, preferably with a sterile dressing. If bleeding continues, apply pressure to the artery that supplies blood to the area. To treat **shock**, place the victim on their back with their legs raised slightly and place a blanket over the body to prevent heat loss. In the case of superficial and partial thickness **burns**, cold water should be applied before dressing with sterile bandages.

flu Abbreviation of INFLUENZA

follicle-stimulating hormone (FSH) Hormone produced by the anterior pituitary gland found in the brain of mammals. In females, it regulates ovulation by stimulating the maturation of immature Graafian follicles in the OVARY. In males, FSH promotes spermatogenesis. FSH is an ingredient in most fertility drugs.

food poisoning Acute illness caused by consumption of food that is itself poisonous or which has become poisoned or contaminated with bacteria. Frequently implicated are SALMONELLA bacteria – found in cattle, pigs, poultry and eggs – and listeria – sometimes found in certain types of cheese. Symptoms include abdominal pain, DIARRHOEA, nausea and vomiting. Treatment includes rest, fluids to prevent dehydration and, possibly, medication. *See also* BOTULISM; GASTROENTERITIS

frostbite Freezing of living body tissue in sub-zero temperatures. Frostbite is an effect of the body's defensive response to intense cold, which is to shut down blood vessels at the extremities in order to preserve warmth at the core of the body. Consequently, it mostly occurs in the face, ears, hands and feet. In superficial frostbite, the affected part turns white and cold: it can be treated by gentle thawing. In deep frostbite, ice crystals form in the tissues. The flesh hardens and sensation is lost. It requires urgent medical treatment. No attempt should be made at rewarming if there is a risk of refreezing, as this results in the death of body tissue (gangrene).

gallstone (cholelithiasis) Hard mass, usually composed of CHOLESTEROL and calcium salts, which forms in the gall bladder. Gallstones may cause severe pain or become lodged in the common bile duct, causing obstructive JAUNDICE or cholecystitis. Treatment is by removal of the stones or of the gall bladder.

gamete Reproductive sex cell that joins with another sex cell to form a new organism. Female gametes (ova) are motionless; male gametes (sperm) often have a tail (flagellum) enabling them to swim to the ovum. All gametes are HAPLOID.

gastric juice Fluid comprising a mixture of substances, including PEPSIN and hydrochloric acid, secreted by glands of the stomach. Its principal function is to break down proteins into polypeptides during digestion.

▶ *Gene replacement therapy (GRT)*

GRT is used to treat severe combined immunodeficiency disease (SCID), where the gene that produces adenosine deaminase (ADA) is missing. As ADA is essential for white blood cell production, this renders the body open to infection. Two retroviruses (1) are introduced into the bone marrow. These have the ability to produce RNA from their DNA (2) using a reverse transcriptase enzyme (3). This DNA is then incorporated into the chromosomes (4). When these chromosomes multiply, new viral RNA, viral proteins and ADA are produced (5). The first two produce more new viruses, while the body uses ADA to produce white blood cells.

gastroenteritis Inflammation of the stomach and intestines causing abdominal pain, diarrhoea and vomiting. It may be caused by infection, food poisoning or allergy. Severe cases can cause dehydration. Treatment includes fluid replacement.

gene replacement therapy (GRT) Medical treatment involving the replacement or alteration of faulty genes by means of GENETIC ENGINEERING. Although first used on humans in 1990, it remains a largely experimental procedure. A healthy gene is packaged into some kind of vector (usually a suitably doctored virus) so that it can be targeted at the affected cells. Initially, gene therapy was restricted to the treatment of hereditary disorders such as CYSTIC FIBROSIS and SICKLE-CELL ANAEMIA. Research is being conducted into its suitability as a method for the treatment of certain cancers. *See also* Genes and Inheritance, pp. 110–111

genetic code Set of rules by which genetic instructions located in a cell's DNA are translated to make the structural proteins that build a cell and the enzymes that control its metabolism. Instructions are 'written' in sections of DNA called genes using bases (adenine (A), cytosine (C), guanine (G) and thymine (T)) as 'letters'. Groups of three bases form codons (e.g. GGC), each of which is 'translated' in the cytoplasm into one of 20 amino acids according to

G

G

◀ *Gout Illustration of a foot, showing a tophus (swelling) due to gout. The tophus is seen at the base of the big toe. The area is red, inflamed and tender. Gout is a disease in which a defect in uric acid metabolism causes an excess of the acid and its salts (sodium urate) to accumulate in the blood and joints. The big toe is commonly affected.*

the code. With 43 (64) possible arrangements of base 'letters' there are sufficient codons to code for the 20 different amino acids. Through the genetic code each gene controls the assembly of a unique protein with a specific sequences of amino acids. *See also* GENOME

genetic engineering Construction of a DNA molecule containing a desired gene. The gene is then introduced into a bacterial, fungal, plant or mammalian cell, so that this cell produces the desired protein. It has been used to produce substances such as human growth hormone, insulin and enzymes for biological washing powder. There are concerns about the ethics of genetic engineering both in human medicine and food technology. *See also* BIOTECHNOLOGY; CLONE

genetics Study of heredity. Geneticists study how the characteristics of an organism depend on its genes, how these characteristics pass down to the next generation and how changes may occur through mutation. A person's behaviour, learning ability and physiology may be explained partly by genetics, although the environment has a considerable influence, too. Gregor Mendel established the basic laws of inheritance. The discovery in 1953 of the structure of DNA by Francis Crick, James Watson and Maurice Wilkins

revealed the molecular basis of heredity. *See also* GENETIC CODE; GENETIC ENGINEERING

genome All the DNA in one set of 23 human chromosomes which contains the genes (instructions) for making a human being. By 2003 scientists working for the Human Genome Project had sequenced all the DNA in a genome to determine the sequence of paired bases. They showed that genes make up just 3% of the DNA; the remaining 97% of the genome is made up of 'junk' DNA which appears to have no function. *See also* GENETICS

geriatrics Branch of medicine that deals with the problems of the elderly.

germ Popular term for an infectious agent. Germs can be bacteria, protists, fungi or viruses. In biology, the term denotes a rudimentary stage in plant growth.

German measles (rubella) Viral disease usually contracted in childhood. Symptoms include a sore throat, slight fever and pinkish rash. Women developing rubella during the first three months of pregnancy risk damage to the fetus. Immunization is recommended for girls who have not had the disease.

glandular fever (infectious mononucleosis) Acute disease, usually of young people, caused by the Epstein-Barr virus. It produces an increased number of white cells (monocytes) in the blood. Symptoms include fever, painful enlargement of the lymph nodes and pronounced lassitude.

glaucoma Incurable condition in which pressure within the eye is increased due to an excess of aqueous humour, the fluid within the chamber. It occurs when normal drainage of fluid is interrupted, posing a threat to vision. Most frequently found in people over the age of 40, glaucoma can be managed with drugs and surgery.

glomerulonephritis Group of kidney disorders featuring damage to the glomeruli (clusters of blood vessels in the kidney nephrons). Chronic forms may progress to kidney failure.

gonorrhoea Sexually transmitted disease (STD) caused by the bacterium *Neisseria gonorrhoeae*, causing inflammation of the genital tract. Symptoms include pain on urination and the passing of pus. Some infected women experience no symptoms. It is treated with antibiotics. If not treated, it may spread, causing sterility, ultimately threatening other organs in the body.

gout Form of ARTHRITIS, featuring an excess of uric acid crystals in the tissues. More common in men, it causes attacks of pain and inflammation in the joints, most often those of the feet or hands. It is treated with anti-inflammatories.

gynaecology Area of medicine concerned with the female reproductive organs. Its study and practice are often paired with OBSTETRICS.

haemoglobin Red-coloured protein present in the ERYTHROCYTES (red blood cells) of vertebrates. It carries oxygen to all cells in the body by combining with it to form oxy-haemoglobin. Oxygen attaches to the haem part of the protein, which contains iron: the globin part is a globular protein.

haemophilia Hereditary BLOOD clotting disorder causing prolonged external or internal bleeding, often without apparent cause. **Haemophilia A** is caused by inability to synthesize blood factor VIII, a substance essential to clotting. This can be managed with injections of factor VIII. The rarer **haemophilia B** is caused by a deficiency of blood factor IX. The gene for both types is passed on almost exclusively from mother to son. Haemophilia A occurs in about 1 baby in 5,000 live births. Haemophilia B is occurs in about 1 in 30,000.

haemorrhage Loss of BLOOD from a damaged vessel. It may be external, flowing from a wound, or internal, as from internal injury or a bleeding ulcer. Blood loss from an artery is most serious, causing shock and death if untreated. Chronic bleeding can lead to ANAEMIA. Internal bleeding is signalled by the appearance of blood in the urine or sputum.

haemostasis Process by which bleeding stops. BLOOD vessels constrict, PLATELETS aggregate and PLASMA coagulates to form filaments of FIBRIN.

hallucination Apparent perception of something that is not actually present. Although they may occur in any of the five senses, auditory hallucinations and visual hallucinations are the most common. While they are usually symptomatic of psychotic disorders, hallucinations may also result from fatigue or emotional upsets and can sometimes be a side-effect of certain drugs.

hallucinogen Drug that causes HALLUCINATIONS. Hallucinogenic drugs, such as mescaline, were used in primitive religious ceremonies. Today, drugs such as LSD are taken illicitly.

haploid Term used to describe a cell that has only one member of each CHROMOSOME pair. All human cells except GAMETES are diploid, having 46 chromosomes. Gametes are haploid, having 23 chromosomes. The body cells of many lower organisms, including algae and single-celled organisms, are haploid. *See also* MEIOSIS

H

harelip Congenital cleft in the upper lip caused by the failure of the two parts of the palate to fuse together. It is a congenital condition, often associated with CLEFT PALATE.

hay fever Seasonal ALLERGY induced by pollens. Symptoms include ASTHMA, itching of the nose and eyes and sneezing. Symptoms are controlled with an ANTIHISTAMINE.

headache Pain felt in the skull. Most frequently caused by stress or tension, it may also signal other diseases, especially if associated with fever. *See also* MIGRAINE

heart attack (myocardial infarction) Death of part of the heart muscle due to the blockage of a coronary artery by a blood clot (thrombosis). It is accompanied by pain in the chest and arm, sweating and vomiting. Modern drugs treat abnormal heart rhythms and dissolve clots in the coronary arteries. **Heart failure** occurs when the heart is unable to pump blood at the rate necessary to supply body tissues and may be due to high BLOOD PRESSURE or CORONARY HEART DISEASE. Symptoms include shortness of breath, OEDEMA and fatigue. Treatment is with a DIURETIC and heart drugs. *See also* ANGINA; ARTERIOSCLEROSIS

heart-lung machine Apparatus used during some surgery to take over the function of the heart and lungs. It consists of a pump to circulate blood around the body and special equipment to add oxygen to the blood and remove carbon dioxide.

heatstroke Condition in which the body temperature rises above 41°C (106°F). It is brought on by extreme heat. In mild cases there may be lassitude and fainting; in severe cases, coma and death may ensue.

Heimlich manoeuvre FIRST AID technique, developed by Dr Henry J Heimlich for relieving blockage in the windpipe. The rescuer uses his or her arms to encircle the choking person's chest from behind, positioning one fist in the space just beneath the breastbone and covering it

H

▲ *Hay fever Artwork depicting hay fever showing pollen grains (yellow/brown) entering the nasal cavity (red, centre) of a sufferer. Pollen grains are released in their billions during plants' reproduction. Some people are sensitized to pollen in the air and have an allergic reaction (rhinitis or pollinosis) whenever they are in contact with it. Symptons are caused by a release of the chemical histamine in the body.*

▶ *Hodgkin's lymphoma*
Coloured SEM of dividing Hodgkin's cells taken from the pleural effusions of a 55-year-old, male patient with 'mixed cellularity Hodgkin's disease'. The cells are grown in tissue culture. Hodgkin's disease is a cancer of the lymphoreticular system – the mediator of non-specific cell defence mechanisms and the immune response. The various cell lines of the system are all subject to cancerous changes. In Hodgkin's disease, the nature of the cell line is unknown, but in the most common form the cell population is mixed. Magnification: ×572.

H

with the other hand. The rescuer then thumps the fist into the person's midriff.

hepatitis Inflammation of the liver, usually due to a generalized infection. Early symptoms include lethargy, nausea, fever and muscle and joint pains. Five hepatitis viruses are known: A, B, C, D and E. The most common single cause is the **hepatitis A** virus (HAV). More serious is infection with the **hepatitis B** virus (HBV), which can lead to chronic inflammation or complete failure of the liver and, in some cases, to liver cancer.

hernia Protrusion of an organ, or part of an organ, through its enclosing wall or connective tissue. Common hernias are a protrusion of an intestinal loop through the umbilicus (umbilical hernia), or protrusion of part of the stomach or oesophagus into the chest cavity (hiatus hernia).

heroin Drug derived from MORPHINE. It produces similar effects to morphine, but acts more quickly and is effective in smaller doses. It is prescribed to relieve pain in terminal illness and severe injuries. Widely used illegally, it is more addictive than morphine and can lead eventually to death. *See also* DRUG ADDICTION

herpes Infectious disease resulting in painful skin sores caused by two varieties of the **Herpes simplex virus** (HSV). HSV 1 typically affects the face, causing cold sores; HSV 2 usually affects the genitals, resulting in the STD genital herpes. Another virus in the herpes family, **Herpes zoster**, is responsible for CHICKENPOX and SHINGLES.

histamine Substance derived from the amino acid histidine, occurring naturally in many plants and in animal tissues and released on tissue injury. It is implicated in allergic reactions that can be treated with ANTIHISTAMINE drugs.

hives (urticaria or nettle rash) Transient, itchy reddish or pale raised skin patches. Hives may be caused by an ALLERGY, by irritants such as sunlight or by stress.

Hodgkin's lymphoma (Hodgkin's disease) Rare type of CANCER causing painless enlargement of the lymph glands, lymphatic tissue and spleen, with subsequent spread to other areas. The cancer targets the B-cells and the T-cells of lymph tissue. It was named after English pathologist Thomas Hodgkin (1798–1866) and its treatment typically consists

145

◀ *Human immunodeficiency virus (HIV) Coloured TEM of HIV viruses budding from a host T-lymphocyte white blood cell. The viruses are here acquiring their viral membrane (red) from the host cell membrane. HIV viruses infect T-cells by injecting viral genetic material into the cell, causing it to form new HIV viruses. These new viruses bud out, damaging the cell membrane. The T-cell may thus die, weakening the body's immune system. Magnification: ×72,000.*

H

of RADIOTHERAPY, surgery, drug therapy or a combination of these. It is curable if caught early.

homeostasis In biology, processes that maintain constant conditions within a cell or organism in response to either internal or external changes.

hormone Chemical substance secreted by living cells. Hormones affect the metabolic activities of cells in other parts of the body. In mammals, glands of the endocrine system secrete hormones directly into the bloodstream. Hormones exercise chemical control of physiological functions, regulating growth, development, sexual functioning, metabolism and (in part) emotional balance. They maintain a delicate equilibrium that is vital to health. The hypothalamus, adjacent to the pituitary gland at the base of the brain, is responsible for overall co-ordination of the secretion of hormones. Most hormones are PROTEINS or STEROIDS. Hormones include THYROXINE, ADRENALINE, INSULIN, OESTROGEN, PROGESTERONE and TESTOSTERONE. See also pp. 56–57

hormone replacement therapy (HRT) Drug therapy given to some older women who are experiencing the MENOPAUSE, or women of any age who have had both overies removed. HRT administers OESTROGEN, or a combination of oestrogen and synthetic PROGESTOGEN, to relieve menopausal symptoms such as hot flushes, fatigue and vaginal dryness caused by decreased secretion of those sex hormones by the ovaries. HRT also gives some protection against heart disease and OSTEOPOROSIS but may slightly increase the risk of developing breast and certain other CANCERS.

human immunodeficiency virus (HIV) Organism that causes ACQUIRED IMMUNE DEFICIENCY SYNDROME (AIDS). A RETROVIRUS identified in 1983, HIV attacks the IMMUNE SYSTEM, leaving the person unable to fight off infection. There are two distinct viruses: **HIV-1**, which has now spread worldwide, and **HIV-2**, which is concentrated almost entirely in West Africa. Both cause AIDS. There are three main means of transmission: from person to person by sexual contact, from mother to baby during birth and by contact with contaminated blood or blood products (for instance, during transfusions or when drug users share needles). People can carry the virus for many years before developing symptoms.

Huntington's disease (Huntington's chorea) Acute degenerative disorder. It is genetically transmitted and generally occurs in early middle age. It is caused by the presence of abnormally large amounts of glutamate and aspartate. Physical symptoms include loss of motor co-ordination. Mental deterioration can take various forms.

hydrocephalus Increased volume of cerebrospinal fluid (CSF) in the brain. A condition that exerts dangerous pressure on brain tissue, it can be due to obstruction or a failure of natural reabsorption. In babies, it is congenital; in adults, it may arise from injury or disease. It is treated by insertion of a shunting system to drain the CSF into the abdominal cavity.

hydrotherapy Use of water within the body or on its surface as a treatment of disease. It is often used in conjunction with PHYSIOTHERAPY.

hyperglycaemia Condition in which the blood-sugar level is abnormally high. It can occur in a number of diseases, most notably DIABETES. See also HYPOGLYCAEMIA

hypersensitivity Condition in which a person reacts excessively to a stimulus. Most hypersensitive reactions are synonymous with an ALLERGY, the commonest being HAY FEVER.

hypertension Persistent high BLOOD PRESSURE. It can damage blood vessels and may increase the risk of stroke or heart disease. See also HYPOTENSION

hyperthermia Abnormally high body temperature, usually defined as being 41°C (105.8°F) or more. It is usually due to overheating (as in HEATSTROKE) or FEVER.

hyperthyroidism Excessive production of thyroid hormone, with enlargement of the thyroid gland (in the neck). Symptoms include protrusion of the eyeballs, rapid heart rate, high blood pressure, accelerated metabolism and weight loss. See also HYPOTHYROIDISM; Endocrine system, pp. 56–57

hyperventilation Rapid breathing that is not brought about by physical exertion. It reduces the carbon dioxide level in the blood, producing dizziness, tin-

gling and tightness in the chest; it may cause loss of consciousness.

hypochondria (hypochondriasis) Neurotic condition characterized by an exaggerated concern with ill health. Hypochondriacs imagine they have serious diseases and often consult several doctors in the hope of a 'cure'.

hypodermic syringe Surgical instrument for injecting fluids beneath the skin into a muscle or blood vessel. It comprises a graduated tube containing a piston plunger, connected to a hollow needle. See also INJECTION

hypoglycaemia Abnormally low level of sugar in the blood. It may result from fasting, excess INSULIN in the blood or various metabolic and glandular diseases, notably DIABETES. Symptoms include dizziness, headache, sweating and mental confusion. See also HYPERGLYCAEMIA

H

▲ *Hypodermic syringe* A collection of syringes and hypodermic needles. Hypodermic syringes are used for administering vital fluids to patients.

hypotension Condition in which BLOOD PRESSURE is abnormally low. It is commonly seen after heavy blood loss or excessive fluid loss due to prolonged vomiting or diarrhoea. It also occurs in many serious illnesses. Temporary hypotension may cause sweating, dizziness and fainting. *See also* HYPERTENSION

hypothermia Fall in body temperature to below 35°C (95°F). Most at risk are newborns and the elderly. Insidious in onset, it can progress to coma and death. Hypothermia is sometimes induced during surgery to lower the body's oxygen demand. It occurs naturally in animals during hibernation.

hypothyroidism Deficient functioning of the thyroid gland. Congenital hypothyroidism can lead to cretinism in children. In adults, the condition is called **myxoedema**. More common in women, it causes physical and mental slowness, weight gain, sensitivity to cold and susceptibility to infection. It can be due to a defect of the gland or a lack of iodine in the diet. It is treated with the hormone thyroxine.

hysterectomy Removal of the uterus, possibly with surrounding structures. It is performed to treat fibroids or cancer or to put an end to heavy menstrual bleeding.

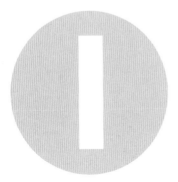

ibuprofen Developed in the 1960s, a type of non-steroidal anti-inflammatory drug (NSAIDs) that is taken to reduce the symptoms of PAIN, FEVER and INFLAMMATION. Other NSAIDs include aspirin.

immune system System by which the body defends itself against disease. It involves many kinds of LEUCOCYTES (white blood cells) in the blood, lymph and bone marrow. Some of the cells (B-cells) make antibodies against invading microbes and other foreign bodies (ANTIGENS) or neutralize TOXINS produced by pathogens, while other antibodies encourage phagocytes and macrophages to attack and digest invaders. T-cells also provide a variety of functions in the immune system. *See also* INTERFERON; Immune system, pp. 72–73

immunity In medicine, protection against or resistance to DISEASE. Genetic factors and general health influence **innate** immunity. **Acquired** immunity is the body's second line of defence. An infecting agent stimulates the IMMUNE SYSTEM to respond to the presence of ANTIGENS. In **cell-mediated** immunity sensitized cells react directly with the antigen. This form of immunity is suppressed by HUMAN IMMUNODEFICIENCY VIRUS (HIV). Immunity may be induced artificially by IMMUNIZATION.

immunization Practice of conferring IMMUNITY against disease by artificial means. Passive immunity may be conferred by the injection of an antiserum containing antibodies. Active immunity involves vaccination with dead or attenuated (weakened) organisms to stimulate production of specific antibodies and so provide lasting immunity. Immunization against certain disease usually begins early in infanthood.

immunoglobulin Protein found in the BLOOD that plays a role in the IMMUNE SYSTEM. Immunoglobulins act as antibodies for specific ANTIGENS. They can be obtained from donor plasma and injected into people at risk of particular diseases.

immunology Study of IMMUNITY and ALLERGY. It is concerned with the prevention of disease by vaccination (**active** immunity) or by injections of antibodies (**passive** immunity). Allergic reactions result from an overactive response to harmless foreign substances such as dust, rather than to infective organisms.

▶ **Influenza** *Coloured TEM of stages of cell infection of an influenza virus. The virus appears rounded, with a core of RNA. It has a spiked outer coat which allows the virus to attach to host cells. In the top frames, the virus attaches to the cell. In the lower frames, the virus penetrates the cell, infecting it and causing more influenza viruses to be produced.*
Magnification: ×50,000.

immunosuppressive drug Any drug that suppresses the body's immune responses to infection or 'foreign' tissue. Such drugs are used to prevent rejection of transplanted organs and to treat autoimmune disease and some cancers. STEROIDS, such as CORTISONE, which suppress lymphocyte cells, have been used in transplants.

impetigo Contagious skin condition caused by *staphylococcus aureus* infection. It causes multiple spreading lesions with yellowish-brown crusts. The bacterium often lives harmlessly inside the nose.

impotence In men, the inability to perform SEXUAL INTERCOURSE through lack of an erection. It may be temporary or permanent, brought about by illness, injury, the effects of certain drugs, fatigue or psychological factors.

incubation period In medicine, the time-lag between becoming infected with a disease and the appearance of the first symptoms. In many infectious diseases, the incubation period is quite short – anything from a few hours to a few days – although it may also be very variable.

indigestion *See* DYSPEPSIA

induction Initiation of LABOUR before it starts naturally. It involves perforating the fetal membranes and administering the hormone oxytocin to stimulate contractions of the uterus. It is undertaken where there is medical risk to the mother or baby in waiting for labour to begin naturally.

infarction Death of part of an organ caused by a sudden obstruction in an artery supplying it. In a myocardial infarction (HEART ATTACK), a section of heart muscle dies.

infection Invasion of the body by disease-causing organisms that become established, multiply and give rise to symptoms.

infertility Inability to reproduce. In a woman it may be due to a failure to ovulate (the release of an ovum for fertilization), obstruction of the Fallopian tube or disease of the ENDOMETRIUM. In a man it is due to inadequate sperm production. *See also* pp. 102–103

inflammation Reaction of body tissue to infection or injury, with resulting pain, heat, swelling and redness. It occurs when damaged cells release HISTAMINE, which causes blood vessels at the damaged site to dilate. LEUCOCYTES invade the area to engulf bacteria. MACROPHAGES remove dead tissue, sometimes with the formation of pus.

influenza Viral infection mainly affecting the airways, with chesty symptoms, headache, joint pains, fever and general malaise. It is treated by bed rest and painkillers. Vaccines are available to confer immunity to some strains.

injection In medicine, use of a syringe and needle to introduce drugs or other fluids into the body to diagnose, treat or prevent disease. Most injections are either **intravenous** (into a vein), **intramuscular** (into a muscle) or **intradermal** (into the skin).

insomnia Inability to sleep. It may be caused by anxiety, pain or stimulants such as drugs.

insulin Hormone secreted by the islets of Langerhans in the pancreas and concerned with the control of blood-glucose levels. Insulin lowers the level of blood-glucose by helping the uptake of glucose into cells, and by causing the liver to convert glucose to glycogen. In the absence of insulin, glucose accumulates in the blood and urine, resulting in DIABETES. In 1921 Frederick Banting and Charles Best isolated insulin. Its structure was discovered by Frederick Sanger. *See also* pp. 56–57 and 88–89

interferon Protein produced by cells when infected with a VIRUS. Interferons can help uninfected cells to resist infection by the virus and may also impede virus replication and protein synthesis. In some circumstances, they can inhibit cell growth. Human interferon is now produced by GENETIC ENGINEERING to treat some CANCERS, HEPATITIS and MULTIPLE SCLEROSIS (MS).

intoxication Condition arising when the body is poisoned by any toxic substance, whether liquid, solid or gas. Symptoms vary according to the ingested substance. The term is most commonly used in connection with alcohol consumption.

intravenous drip Apparatus for delivering drugs, blood and blood products, nutrients and other fluids directly into the bloodstream. A hollow needle is inserted into an appropriate vein and then attached to tubing leading from a bag containing the solution.

in vitro fertilization (IVF) Use of artificial techniques to join an ovum with sperm outside (*in vitro*) a woman's body to help infertile couples to have children of their own. The basic technique of IVF involves removing ova from a woman's ovaries, fertilizing them in the laboratory and then inserting them into her uterus. In **zygote intrafallopian transfer (ZIFT)**, a fertilized egg (zygote) is returned to the fallopian tube, from which it makes its own way to the uterus. The zygote then divides to form an embryo. In **gamete intrafallopian transfer (GIFT)**, the ova are removed, mixed with sperm and then both ova and sperm are inserted into a fallopian tube to be fertilized in the natural setting. The first 'test-tube baby', Louise Joy Brown, was born in England in

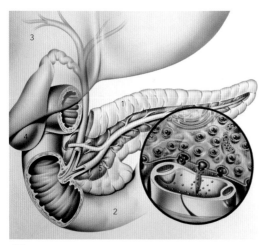

◄ *Insulin* Artwork of the human pancreas showing production of the hormone insulin. The pancreas (*1*) is a tapered gland situated in the loop of the duodenum (*2*) and below the liver (*3*) and gall bladder (*4*). The pancreas has both digestive and hormonal functions. Its exocrine tissue produces digestive enzymes which pass into the intestine through the pancreatic duct (*5*). Production of the hormone insulin by the endocrine pancreas is shown inset. A beta cell (**red**) contained within an islet of Langerhans secretes insulin (**blue**) into a capillary (**grey**).

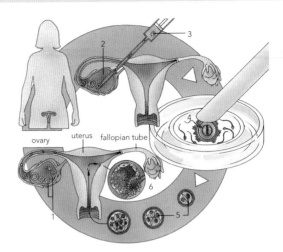

► *In vitro fertilization* This technique was developed to help women who are unable to conceive. The mother, or egg donor, is given hormone treatment to cause many ovarian follicles to develop (*1*). While the ovary is observed through a laparoscope, a needle (*2*) is inserted into each follicle, which is then transferred (*3*) to a petri dish where sperm are added (*4*). As the zygote divides (*5*) to 16 cells, it is introduced into the uterus through a plastic tube so that it can implant in the wall (*6*) and progress normally.

ovary   uterus   fallopian tube

1978. *See also* INFERTILITY; Fertilization and Implantation, pp. 102–103

IVF Abbreviation of IN VITRO FERTILIZATION

effects on physiological and psychological rhythms. Symptoms include fatigue, confusion, mood alterations, irritability, sleep disturbance and other signs of stress.

jaundice Yellowing of the skin and the whites of the eyes, caused by an excess of BILE pigment in the blood. Mild jaundice is common in newborn babies. In adults, jaundice may occur when the flow of bile from the liver to the intestine is blocked by an obstruction such as a GALL-STONE or in diseases such as CIRRHOSIS, HEPATITIS and ANAEMIA.

jet lag Phenomenon experienced when the body clock is disrupted by the sudden change in time zones, causing adverse

keratin Fibrous protein present in large amounts in skin cells, where it serves as a protective layer. Hair and fingernails are made up of cells filled with keratin.

kidney machine (artificial kidney) Equipment designed to remove toxic wastes from the blood in kidney failure. Plastic tubing is used to pipe blood from the body into the machine, where waste products are filtered out by DIALYSIS. In 1943 the first kidney machine was built by Dutch physician Willem Kolff.

hormone oxytocin controls the propulsion of milk from the breast.

lactose (milk sugar) Disaccharide present in milk, made up of a molecule of glucose linked to a molecule of galactose.

laryngitis Inflammation of the larynx and vocal cords. Symptoms include a sore throat, hoarseness, coughing and breathing difficulties. It is usually due to a respiratory tract infection but may also be caused by exposure to irritant gases or chemicals. *See also* Larynx and Speech, pp. 80–81

labour In childbirth, stage in the delivery of the fetus at the end of PREGNANCY. In the first stage, contractions of the uterus begin, the cervix dilates in readiness and the sac containing the amniotic fluid ruptures. In the second stage, the contractions strengthen and the baby is propelled through the birth canal. The third stage is the expulsion of the placenta and fetal membranes, together known as the afterbirth. *See also* Childbirth, pp. 106–107

laser surgery Surgery carried out using a laser. The high energy in an narrow laser beam can burn through body tissues to make a fine 'cut'. The heat also seals blood vessels, so there is less bleeding than when a knife is used. Less powerful lasers can remove marks from the skin. Some forms of skin cancer are treated in this way. Laser surgery is also used to reshape the cornea at the front of the eye in order to restore normal, focused vision to people suffering from MYOPIA.

lactation Secretion of milk to feed the young. In pregnant women, hormones induce the breasts to enlarge and PROLACTIN stimulates mammary glands to begin secreting milk. The milk appears in the breast after the birth of the baby. The

Lassa fever Acute viral disease, classified as a haemorrhagic fever. The virus, first detected in 1969, is spread by a species of rat found only in West Africa. It is characterized by internal bleeding, with fever, headache and muscle pain.

◄ *Lactose Polarized light micrograph (PLM) of crystals of the sugar lactose found in milk. Lactose is a white sugar occurring in solution in the milk of all mammals. Human milk contains 6% lactose while cow's milk contains 4%. Lactose is commercially prepared by evaporation of the whey obtained in cheesemaking. Like table sugar (sucrose), it is a disaccharide consisting of two basic sugar units: glucose and galactose. Magnification: ×63.*

► **Leucocyte** Coloured SEM of a leucocyte (white blood cell) surrounded by Staphylococcus aureus bacteria. The leucocyte (mauve) is part of the body's defence against the presence of the bacteria (red).
Magnification: ×5,500.

laxative Agent used to counteract constipation. Various kinds are available, including bulk-forming drugs, stimulant laxatives, faecal softeners and saline purgatives.

L-dopa (levodopa) Naturally occurring amino acid used to relieve some symptoms of PARKINSON'S DISEASE. It sometimes suppresses the trembling, unsteadiness and slowness of movement that characterize the condition.

legionnaire's disease Lung disease caused by infection with the bacterium *Legionella pneumophila*. It takes its name from the serious outbreak that occurred during a convention of the American Legion held in Philadelphia, USA, in 1976. The bacterium thrives in water and may be found in defective heating, ventilation and air-conditioning systems. It is inhaled in fine water droplets present in the air.

Leishmaniasis Insect-borne disease carrying a high mortality and caused by infection with the parasite *Leishmania donovani*, transmitted by sandflies. The spleen is particularly affected and becomes enlarged. Symptoms include fever, anaemia and wasting. The disease occurs primarily in the Mediterranean region, Africa, Asia and Central and South America.

leprosy (Hansen's disease) Chronic, progressive condition affecting the skin and nerves, caused by infection with the microorganism *Mycobacterium leprae*. There are two main forms. **Lepromatous** leprosy is a contagious form in which raised nodules appear on the skin and there is thickening of the skin and peripheral nerves. In **tuberculoid** leprosy, there is loss of sensation in parts of the skin, sometimes with loss of pigmentation and hair. Now confined almost entirely to the tropics, leprosy can be treated with a combination of drugs, but the nerve damage is irreversible.

leucocyte (white BLOOD cell) Colourless structure with a nucleus and cytoplasm. The three types are LYMPHOCYTES, monocytes and granulocytes. Normal blood contains 5,000–10,000 of them per cu mm (0.000035 fl oz). Excessive numbers of leucocytes are seen in such diseases as LEUKAEMIA. *See also* PHAGOCYTE; IMMUNE SYSTEM

leukaemia One of a group of cancers of the bone marrow and other blood-forming tissues that results in the proliferation of abnormal, immature LEUCOCYTES (white blood cells) that remain unspecialized and functionless. These cells crowd out and suppress production of normal red and white blood cells and platelets resulting in infection, ANAEMIA and bleeding problems. Leukaemias are classified according to the abnormal cell type involved. Lymphoblastic (lymphocytic) leukaemia involves the cell line that produces LYMPHOCYTES, while myelogenous (myelocytic) leukaemia involves

L

◀ *Leukaemia* Illustration of chronic myelogenous leukaemia showing an abnormal proliferation of immature granulocytes in the bloodstream.

the cell line that gives rise to granulocytes such as neutrophils. Acute leukaemia advances rapidly and derives from very immature leucocytes; chronic leukaemia takes months or years to progress and involves more mature leucocytes. The four forms are: acute lymphoblastic leukaemia (ALL), the most common form in children; acute myelogenous leukaemia (AML); chronic lymphoblastic leukaemia (CLL), mostly in older adults, and chronic myelogenous leukaemia (CML). Without treatment such as RADIOTHERAPHY and CHEMOTHERAPY all leukaemias, whether acute or chronic, are fatal: only the timescale differs.

long-sightedness (hyperopia) Defect of vision that causes distant objects to be seen more clearly than nearby ones. In a long-sighted person, the focusing distance of the eyeball is too short and, as a result, light rays entering the eye strike the retina before they can be properly focused. Long-sightedness is corrected by convex lenses. *See also* MYOPIA

lumbago Pain in the lower (lumbar) region of the back. It is usually due to strain or poor posture. When associated with SCIATICA, it may be due to a SLIPPED DISC. *See also* RHEUMATISM

lupus erythematosus Autoimmune disease affecting the skin and connective tissue. The discoid form causes red patches covered with scales, often on the cheeks and nose. The systemic or disseminated form varies in severity. Nine times more common in women than in men, the disease is treated mainly with corticosteroids.

lyme disease Condition caused by a spirochete (spiral-shaped bacterium) transmitted by the bite of a tick that lives on deer. It usually begins with a red rash, often accompanied by fever, headache and pain in the muscles and joints. Untreated, the disease can lead to chronic arthritis and there may also be involvement of the nervous system, heart, liver or kidneys. It is treated with ANTIBIOTICS.

lymph node One of many bean-shaped swellings occurring along lymph vessels. It contains a network of fibres and white blood cells, including MACROPHAGES and LYMPHOCYTES, that filter out and destroy pathogens, malignant cells and debris from the lymph that flows through it. *See also* Lymphatic system, pp. 70-71

lymphocyte Type of LEUCOCYTE (white blood cell) in vertebrates. Produced in bone marrow, they are mostly found in the lymph and blood and around infected sites. In human beings, lymphocytes form c.25% of white blood cells and play an important role in combating disease. **B-lymphocytes** produce antibodies and **T-lymphocytes** maintain IMMUNITY. *See also* ANTIBODY

L

site and also used as an antacid, is often also called magnesia.

magnetic resonance imaging (MRI) Diagnostic scanning system, based on the use of powerful magnets, which produces images of soft tissues in the body. Magnetic resonance imaging (MRI) is invaluable for producing images of the brain and spinal cord in particular. The scanner's magnet causes the nuclei within the atoms of the patient's body to line themselves up in one direction. A brief radio pulse is then beamed at the nuclei, causing them to spin. As they realign themselves to the magnet, they give off weak radio signals that can be recorded and converted electronically into images.

malaria Parasitic disease resulting from infection with one of four species of *Plasmodium* protist (unicellular organism). Transmitted by the *Anopheles* mosquito, it is characterized by fever and enlargement of the spleen. Attacks of fever, chills and sweating typify the disease and recur as new generations of parasites develop in the blood. The original antimalarial drug, malarone, gave way to synthetics such as chloroquine. With 500 million people infected, malaria is one of

macrophage Large LEUCOCYTE (white blood cell) found wandering in the tissues and fixed in the liver, spleen and lymph nodes. It engulfs pathogens by phagocytosis. Working together with lymphocytes, it forms part of the immune system.

mad cow disease Popular name for BOVINE SPONGIFORM ENCEPHALOPATHY (BSE)

magnesia Magnesium oxide (MgO), a white, neutral, stable powder formed when magnesium burns in oxygen. It is used medicinally in stomach powders. **Magnesium carbonate**, found as magne-

▶ *Malaria An infected mosquito injects thousands of* Plasmodium *organisms into the bloodstream when it bites a human (1). These penetrate liver cells, multiply and cause cell rupture (2). Organisms may re-infect liver cells (3), but usually progress to infect red blood cells (4, 5). Male and female parasites appear in the red blood cells (6). Another mosquito bites the human and takes infected blood (7). Fertilization occurs within the mosquito, the 'embryo' penetrating the stomach wall (8). The cycle continues (9).*

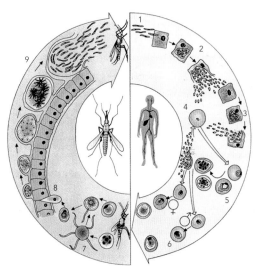

M

the most widespread diseases, claiming up to 2.5 million lives a year.

malnutrition Condition resulting from a diet that is deficient in components such as proteins, fats or carbohydrates. It can lead to deficiency diseases, increased vulnerability to infection and death. *See also* FAMINE

manic depression (bipolar disorder) Mental illness featuring recurrent bouts of depression, possibly alternating with periods of mania. Depressive and manic symptoms may alternate in a cyclical pattern, be mixed or be separated by periods of remission and disturbances of thought and judgement.

mastectomy In surgery, removal of all or part of the female breast. It is performed to treat CANCER. **Simple** mastectomy involves the breast alone. If the cancer has spread, **radical** mastectomy may be undertaken, removing also the lymphatic tissue from the armpit.

ME (**m**yalgic **e**ncephalomyelitis) Condition defined as extreme fatigue that persists for six months or more. Also known as **chronic fatigue syndrome** or **post-viral fatigue syndrome**, it may be accompanied by other non-specific symptoms, such as fever, headache, muscle and joint pains, dizziness and mood changes. Often occurring after a VIRUS infection, it ranges in severity from chronic weariness to total physical collapse. The cause of ME is unknown.

measles (rubeola) Extremely infectious viral disease of children. The symptoms (fever, catarrh, skin rash and spots inside the mouth) appear about two weeks after exposure. Hypersensitivity to light is characteristic. Complications such as pneumonia occasionally occur and middle-ear infection is also a hazard. Vaccination produces life-long IMMUNITY.

medicine Practice of the prevention, diagnosis and treatment of disease or injury: the term also applies to any agent used in the treatment of disease. Medicine has been practised since ancient times, but the dawn of modern Western medicine coincided with accurate anatomical and physiological observations first made in the 17th century. By the 19th century, practical diagnostic procedures had been developed for many diseases: BACTERIA had been discovered and research undertaken for the production of immunizing serums in attempts to eradicate disease. The great developments of the 20th century included the discovery of PENICILLIN and INSULIN, CHEMOTHERAPY (the treatment of various diseases with specific chemical agents), new surgical procedures including organ transplants and sophisticated diagnostic

◀ *Measles Coloured TEM of measles viruses budding off the surface of an infected cell (bottom, pink/yellow). The lipoprotein envelopes of the viruses (red) surround the nucleocapsid (blue). The envelopes are acquired from the host cell's cytoplasmic membrane as the viruses bud from the surface. They enclose the nucleocapsid: a helical structure consisting of a single-stranded RNA core surrounded by protein. Measles is very infectious and mainly affects children. Magnification: ×14,400.*

M

► *Meningitis Coloured MRI scan of a section through the head of a 34-year-old woman. The brain is seen, with the folded cerebrum (at top), brainstem (centre) and cerebellum (centre right). The spinal cord passes into the neck. Meningitis infection is coloured yellow on surfaces of the brain and spinal cord. Meningitis is an inflammation of the meninges – the membranes that cover and protect the brain and spinal cord. It is caused by either bacterial or viral infection.*

devices such as radioactive TRACERS and scanners. Alternative therapies, such as OSTEOPATHY, homeopathy or ACUPUNCTURE, some of which are hundreds of years old, are becoming increasingly popular, and some therapies are being accepted within conventional medicine.

meiosis The process of cell division that reduces the CHROMOSOME number from DIPLOID to HAPLOID. The first division halves the chromosome number in the cells; the second then forms four haploid 'daughter' cells, each containing a unique configuration of the parent cells' chromosomes. In the majority of higher organisms, the resulting haploid cells are the GAMETES, ova and sperm. In this way, meiosis enables the genes from both parents to combine in a single cell without increasing the overall number of chromosomes. *See also* MITOSIS

melanin Dark pigment found in the skin, hair and parts of the eye. The amount of melanin determines skin colour. Absence of melanin results in an ALBINO.

melanoma Type of skin CANCER. They are highly malignant tumours formed by melanocytes, cells in the skin that make the dark pigment MELANIN. They may also occur in mucous membranes and in the eye. Untreated, they may spread to the

liver and lymph nodes. Excessive exposure to sunlight has been cited as a causative factor. Treatment is usually by surgery.

Menière's disease Chronic condition of the inner ear affecting hearing and balance. Symptoms include deafness, vertigo and ringing in the ears (tinnitus). Caused by an excessive amount of fluid in the inner ear, it usually occurs in middle age or later. It is generally treated with ANTIHISTAMINE drugs.

meningitis Inflammation of the **meninges** (membranes) covering the brain and spinal cord, resulting from infection by bacteria or viruses. **Bacterial meningitis** is less common but more serious than its viral counterpart. The germs live naturally at the back of the nose and throat of one in ten people and can be spread by close prolonged contact. Symptoms include headache, fever, nausea and stiffness of the neck. The disease can vary from mild to lethal.

menopause Stage in a woman's life marking the end of her reproductive years, when ovulation and menstruation finally cease, generally around the age of 50. It may be accompanied by side-effects such as hot flushes, excessive bleeding and emotional upset. Hormone replacement

M

◀ *Multiple sclerosis (MS)* Illustration of the brain and spinal cord of a woman suffering from MS. Also seen is a magnified view of the spinal cord showing nerve fibres (*1*). At lower right is a magnified view of an axon within one of the nerve fibres covered with a protective myelin sheath. In MS, patches of the myelin sheath are destroyed. These patches of destroyed myelin are known as plaques (*2*). The damaged fibres affect nerve impulses.

therapy (HRT) is designed to relieve menopausal symptoms.

menstrual cycle Series of events, repeated monthly and affecting the female reproductive system, in which the body prepares for pregnancy. In humans, the average cycle is 28 days. At the beginning of the cycle, hormones from the pituitary gland stimulate the growth of an ovum contained in a follicle in one of the two ovaries. At approximately mid-cycle, the follicle bursts, the ovum releases (**ovulation**) and travels down the FALLOPIAN TUBE to the uterus. The follicle (now called the **corpus luteum**) secretes two hormones, PROGESTERONE and OESTROGEN, during this secretory phase and the ENDOMETRIUM thickens, ready to receive the fertilized ovum. If fertilization (conception) does not occur, the corpus luteum degenerates, hormone secretion ceases, the endometrium breaks down and menstruation occurs in the form of a loss of blood. In the event of conception, the corpus luteum remains and maintains the endometrium with hormones until the placenta is formed. In humans, the onset of the menstrual cycle occurs at PUBERTY and ceases with the MENOPAUSE (around 50 years of age). *See also* pp. 100–103

metabolism Chemical and physical processes and changes continuously occurring in an organism. These processes include the breakdown of organic matter (**catabolism**), resulting in energy release and the synthesis of organic components (**anabolism**) to store energy and build and repair tissues. *See also* RESPIRATION

microbiology Study of microorganisms, their structure, function and significance. Mainly concerned with VIRUSES and single cell forms such as bacteria, protists and fungi, it has immense applications in medicine and the food industry. Microbiology began in the 17th century with the invention of the microscope, which enabled scholars to view microorganisms for the first time. Pioneers include Robert Hooke, Anton van Leeuwenhoek and Louis Pasteur.

microsurgery Delicate surgery performed under a binocular microscope using specialized instruments, such as microneedles as small as 2 mm (0.08 in) long, ENDOSCOPES and lasers. It is used in a number of specialized areas, including the repair of nerves and blood vessels; eye, ear and brain surgery and the reattachment of severed parts.

migraine Recurrent attacks of throbbing headache, mostly on one side only, often accompanied by nausea, vomiting and visual disturbances. It results from changes in diameter of the arteries serving the brain. More common in women, it is seen usually in young adults and may often run in families. Attacks, which may last anything from two to 72 hours, are often associated with trigger factors, such as certain foods (especially chocolate), missed meals, consumption of alcohol, fatigue, exposure to bright light and use of the contraceptive pill. It can be treated, or in some cases prevented, with various drugs.

mineral In NUTRITION, naturally occuring substance that is an important dietary element. The 'major' minerals are calcium and phosphorus as they are required in large amounts, particularly to aid growth of teeth and bones. '**Trace**' minerals are needed in tiny amounts and include iron, sodium, chlorine, sulphur, zinc, copper, manganese and magnesium. All minerals are consumed in a well-balanced diet. *See also* VITAMIN

minimal access surgery Operations that do not involve cutting open the body in the traditional way. Minimal access (**keyhole**) procedures are performed either by means of an ENDOSCOPE or by passing miniature instruments through a fine catheter into a large blood vessel. The surgical laser is also used.

miscarriage Common term for a spontaneous ABORTION, the loss of a fetus from the uterus

mitosis Cell division resulting in two genetically identical 'daughter' cells with the same number of chromosomes as the parent cell. Mitosis is the normal process of tissue growth and is also involved in asexual reproduction. *See also* MEIOSIS

mononucleosis, infectious *See* GLANDULAR FEVER

morphine White, crystalline alkaloid derived from OPIUM. It depresses the CENTRAL NERVOUS SYSTEM and is used as an ANALGESIC for severe pain. An addictive drug, its use is associated with a number of side-effects, including nausea. Morphine was first isolated in 1806. *See also* HEROIN

multiple sclerosis (MS) Incurable disorder of unknown cause in which there is degeneration of the myelin sheath that surrounds nerves in the brain and spinal cord. Striking mostly young adults, symptoms may include unsteadiness, loss of co-ordination and speech and visual disturbances. MS sufferers typically have relapses and remissions over many years.

mumps Viral disease, most common in children, characterized by fever, pain and swelling of one or both parotid salivary glands (located just in front of the ears). The symptoms are more serious in adults and in men inflammation of the testes (orchitis) may occur, with the risk of sterility.

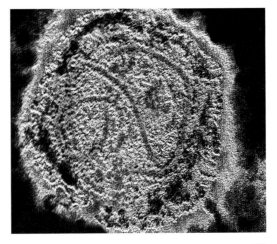

▶ *Mumps Coloured TEM of a section through a mumps virus in a capsule. The long, thin chains (red) contain ribonucleic acid (RNA) genetic material. They are seen in a capsule (pink). The mumps virus is a paramyxovirus. The infection usually causes swelling of the parotid glands of the neck. It is a common childhood disease and symptoms normally subside within three days.*

M

muscular dystrophy Any of a group of hereditary disorders in which the characteristic feature is progressive weakening and ATROPHY of the muscles. Muscle fibres degenerate, to be replaced by fatty tissue. The most common type, **Duchenne muscular dystrophy**, affects about one male infant in 3,000. There is a milder form called **Becker's muscular dystrophy**, which develops in young adults.

myopia (short-sightedness) Common disorder of vision in which near objects are seen sharply, but distant objects are hazy. It is caused either by the eyeball being too long or the eye's lens being too powerful, so light rays entering the eye focus in front of the retina. It is easily corrected with concave lenses in spectacles or contact lenses.

myxoedema Disease caused by deficient function of the thyroid gland, resulting in fatigue, constipation, dry skin, a tendency towards weight gain and, in the later stages, a dulling of mental lucidity. It mostly affects middle-aged women. Treatment involves the administration of the thyroid hormone thyroxine. *See also* pp. 56–57

narcotic Any drug that induces sleep and/or relieves pain. The term is used especially in relation to OPIUM and its derivatives. These drugs have largely been replaced as sedatives because of their addictive properties, but they are still used for severe pain, notably in terminal illness. Other narcotics include alcohols and BARBITURATES.

National Health Service (NHS) In Britain, system of state provision of health care established in 1948. The NHS undertook to provide free, comprehensive coverage for most health services, including hospitals, general medical practice and public health facilities. It is administered by the Department of Health. General practitioners (GPs) have registered patients. They may also have private patients and may contract out of the state scheme altogether. They refer patients, when necessary, to specialist consultants in hospitals. Health visitors, such as midwives and district nurses, are the third arm of the service. Hospitals are administered by regional boards. In 1990, the Conservative government introduced the concept of the 'internal market' into health care, establishing GP fund-holding practices and NHS Trusts independent of local health authority control. In 1997, the Labour government announced that it would replace the internal market with primary care groups consisting of GPs and community nurses. The NHS is the largest employer in the UK.

naturopathy Alternative therapy that relies exclusively on the use of natural treatments, such as exposure to sunlight, fresh air and a healthy diet of organically grown foods. People practising naturopathy prefer the use of herbal remedies to manufactured drugs.

necrosis Death of tissue. It can be caused by disease, injury or interference with the blood supply.

nephritis Inflammation of the kidney. It is a general term used to describe a condition rather than any specific disease. It can progress to kidney failure.

nervous breakdown Popular term for a mental and emotional crisis in which the person either is unable or feels unable to function normally. It is an imprecise term and refers to any of a range of conditions. Nervous breakdowns are usually caused by periods of extreme emotional stress.

neuralgia Intense pain from a damaged nerve, possibly tracking along its course.

► *Neurotransmitter Coloured SEM showing the junction sites, also known as synapses, between nerve fibres and a nerve cell grown in culture. Two nerve fibres coloured purple run diagonally. At top is the surface of a nerve cell (yellow), to which the nerve fibres have formed synapses. Impulses travel down these fibres into the nerve cell, typical of dendrites. The fibres branch before forming their junctions, which appear as terminal swellings (top left). Across these swellings neurotransmitter chemicals pass into the cell in response to nerve fibre impulses and in this way the cell is stimulated. Magnification: ×10,000.*

Forms include trigeminal neuralgia, which features attacks of stabbing pain in the mouth area, and post-herpetic neuralgia following an attack of SHINGLES.

neurology Branch of medicine dealing with the diagnosis and treatment of diseases of the nervous system. *See also* Nervous system, pp. 34–55

neurosis Emotional disorder such as anxiety, depression or various phobias. It is a form of mental illness in which the main disorder is of mood, but the person does not lose contact with reality as happens in PSYCHOSIS.

neurotransmitter Any one of several dozen chemicals involved in communication between neurons or between a nerve and muscle cells. When an electrical impulse arrives at a nerve ending, a neurotransmitter is released to carry the signal across the synapse (specialized junction) between the nerve cell and its neighbour. Some drugs work by disrupting neurotransmission. *See also* pp. 34–55

nicotine Poisonous alkaloid obtained from the leaves of tobacco, used in agriculture as a pesticide and in veterinary medicine to kill external parasites. Nicotine is the principal addictive agent in smoking tobacco. *See also* ADDICTION

nitroglycerine Oily liquid used in medicine (as glyceryl trinitrate) to relieve the symptoms of ANGINA.

noradrenaline Hormone secreted by nerves in the autonomic nervous system and by the adrenal glands (on top of the kidneys). It slows the heart rate and constricts small arteries, thus raising the blood pressure. It is used therapeutically to combat the fall in blood pressure that accompanies SHOCK.

nursing Profession that has as its general function the care of people who – through ill health, disability, immaturity or advanced age – are unable to care for themselves. The Christian Church emphasized caring for the sick, and many religious orders performed such 'acts of mercy'. In the 19th century, Florence Nightingale revealed the need for reforms in nursing and by the end of the century, Britain and the United States had adopted some of her principles. Modern nursing provides a broad range of services, with standards set by relevant professional bodies.

nutrition Process by which humans obtain nutrients from food and the science which deals with food. The science of nutrition involves identifying the kinds and amounts of nutrients necessary for growth and health. Nutrients are generally divided into PROTEINS, CARBOHYDRATES, FATS, MINERALS and VITAMINS. *See also* DIET

O

obesity Condition of being overweight, generally defined as weighing 20% or more above the recommended norm for the person's sex, height and build. People who are overweight are at increased risk of disease and have a shorter life expectancy than those of normal weight.

obstetrics Branch of medicine that deals with pregnancy, childbirth and the care of women following delivery.

occupational therapy Development of practical skills to assist patients recovering from illness or injury. Therapists oversee a variety of pursuits, from the activities of daily living (ADLs), such as washing and dressing, to hobbies and crafts.

odontology Study of the structure, development and diseases of the teeth. It is closely allied with DENTISTRY.

oedema Abnormal accumulation of fluid in the tissues: it may be generalized or confined to one part, such as the ankles. It may be due to heart failure, obstruction of one or more veins or the increased permeability of the capillary walls.

oestrogen Female sex hormone. First produced by a girl at PUBERTY, oestrogen leads to the development of secondary sexual characteristics: breasts, body hair and redistributed fat. It regulates the MENSTRUAL CYCLE and prepares the uterus for pregnancy. It is also a constituent of the contraceptive PILL. *See* pp. 100–101

onchocerciasis (river blindness) Tropical disease of the skin and connective tissue, caused by infection with filarial worms; it may also affect the eyes, causing blindness. It is transmitted by blood-sucking blackflies found in Central and South America and Africa.

oncogene Gene that, by inducing a cell to divide abnormally, contributes to the development of CANCER. Oncogenes arise from gene mutations (proto-oncogenes), which are present in all normal cells and in some viruses.

oncology Specialty concerned with the diagnosis and treatment of CANCER.

ophthalmology Branch of medicine that specializes in the diagnosis and treatment of diseases of the eye.

▶ *Opium Coloured X-ray of the seed capsule of an opium poppy,* Papaver somniferum. *This is the structure from which opium is collected: the circumference of the capsule is slit, allowing a milky latex to ooze out. The latex hardens to form a plastic gummy substance on exposure to air, which is scraped off and formed into balls.*

▶ *Osteoporosis Coloured SEM of fractured bone tissue from a patient suffering from osteoporosis (brittle bone disease). Osteoporosis causes a reduction in overall bone mass and an increase in the bone's porosity, making it more brittle and likely to fracture. It commonly affects the elderly and post-menopausal women, who experience a decrease in levels of the hormone oestrogen. It may develop after injury or infection.*

ophthalmoscope Instrument for examining the interior of the eye, invented by Hermann von Helmholtz in 1851.

opium Drug derived from the unripe seed pods of the opium poppy. Its components and derivatives have been used as NARCOTICS and ANALGESICS for many centuries. It produces drowsiness and euphoria and reduces pain. MORPHINE and CODEINE are opium derivatives.

optometry Testing of vision in order to prescribe corrective eyewear, such as spectacles or contact lenses. It is distinct from OPHTHALMOLOGY.

orgasm Physiological culmination of sexual stimulation, marked by general release of muscular tension and waves of contractions causing climactic spasms of vaginal muscles in the female and ejaculation (the release of SEMEN) in the male.

orthodontics See DENTISTRY

orthopaedics Branch of medicine that deals with the diagnosis and treatment of diseases, disorders and injuries of bones, muscles, tendons and ligaments.

osteomyelitis Infection of the bone, sometimes spreading along the marrow cavity. Rare except in diabetics, it can arise from a compound fracture, where the bone breaks through the skin, or from infection elsewhere in the body. It is accompanied by fever, swelling and pain. The condition may be treated with immobilization, ANTIBIOTICS and surgical drainage.

osteopathy System of alternative medical treatment based on the use of physical manipulation of joints to rectify damage caused by mechanical stresses.

osteoporosis Condition where there is loss of bone substance, resulting in brittle bones. It is common in older people, especially in women after the MENOPAUSE. It may also occur as a side-effect of prolonged treatment with corticosteroid drugs. There is no cure, but it may be treated with calcium supplements. HORMONE REPLACEMENT THERAPY (HRT) may help to prevent its occurence in post-menopausal women.

otosclerosis Inherited condition in which overgrowth of bone in the middle ear causes deafness. It is gradual in onset and twice as common in women as in men. Surgery can rebuild the sound conduction mechanism.

oxygen debt Insufficient supply of oxygen in the muscles following vigorous exercise. This reduces the breakdown of food molecules that generate energy, causing the muscles to overproduce lactic acid creating a sensation of fatigue and sometimes muscular cramp.

oxytocin Hormone produced by the pituitary gland in women during pregnancy. It stimulates the muscles of the uterus, initiating the onset of labour and maintaining contractions during childbirth. It also stimulates lactation. *See also* pp. 58–59 and 104–105

P

pacemaker (sino-atrial node) Specialized group of cells in the heart that generates impulses that set the pace for the heartbeat. If it fails, it can be replaced by an artificial pacemaker – an electronic unit that stimulates the heart by means of tiny electrical impulses.

paediatrics Medical speciality devoted to the diagnosis and treatment of disease and injury in children. Specialists in this field require a thorough knowledge not only of a wide range of conditions peculiar

to children, but also of normal childhood development and the ways in which it may affect treatment and recovery.

pain Unpleasant sensation signalling actual or threatened tissue damage as a result of illness or injury: it can be **acute** (severe but short-lived) or **chronic** (persisting for a long time). Pain is felt when specific nerve endings are stimulated. Pain is treated in a number of ways, most commonly by drugs known as ANALGESICS.

pap test *See* CERVICAL SMEAR

paracetamol ANALGESIC drug that lessens pain and is also effective in reducing fever. It is used to treat mild to moderate pain, such as headaches, toothaches and rheumatic conditions, and is particularly effective against musculoskeletal pain.

paralysis Weakness or loss of muscle power: it can vary from a mild condition to complete loss of function and sensation in the affected part. It can be associated with almost any disorder of the nervous system, including brain or spinal cord injury, infection, stroke, poisoning or progressive conditions such as a tumour or motor neurone disease. Paralysis is rarely total.

paraplegia PARALYSIS of both legs. It is usually due to spinal cord injury and is

◀ *Pacemaker Coloured chest X-ray showing a surgically implanted heart pacemaker (at upper right). The pacemaker supplies electrical impulses along a lead to the heart to keep it beating regularly. Pacemakers are fitted in patients with a malfunctioning sino-atrial node, the part of the heart which initiates each heartbeat, or in patients with a heart block which impairs the nerve impulses generated by the node. Heart pacemakers may provide a regular impulse or discharge only when a heartbeat is missed.*

▶ *Parasite* Light micrograph (LM) of a cercaria of the fluke Schistosoma haematobium, the cause of the disease schistosomiasis (bilharzia). This cercarial stage lives in lakes and rivers, and penetrates the skin of humans in the water. It matures to the adult form, then migrates to the veins surrounding the bladder. Here the females lay eggs which pass out in the urine and contaminate the local water supply.

P

often accompanied by loss of sensation below the site of the damage.

parasite Organism that lives on or in another organism (the host) upon which it depends for its survival: this arrangement may be harmful to the host. A parasite that lives in the host, such as a schistosome fluke, is called an **endoparasite**. A parasite that survives on the host's exterior, such as a tick, is known as an **ectoparasite**.

Parkinson's disease Degenerative brain disorder characterized by tremor, muscular rigidity and poverty of movement and facial expression. It arises from a lack of the NEUROTRANSMITTER, dopamine. Slightly more common in men, it is rare before the age of 50. Foremost among the drugs used to control the disease is L-DOPA.

pathology Study of diseases, their causes and the changes they produce in the cells, tissues and organs of the body.

pellagra Disease caused by a deficiency of nicotinic acid, one of the B group of VITAMINS. Its symptoms are lesions of the skin and mucous membranes, diarrhoea and mental disturbance.

penicillin ANTIBIOTIC agent derived from moulds of the genus *Penicillium*. Sir Alexander Fleming discovered penicillin, the first antibiotic, in 1928. It was synthesized and first became available in 1941. Penicillin was widely used for treating casu-

alties in World War II. It can produce allergic reactions and some microorganisms have become resistant.

pepsin Digestive enzyme secreted by glands of the stomach wall as part of the GASTRIC JUICE. In the presence of hydrochloric acid, it catalyses the splitting of proteins in food into polypeptides. *See* pp. 86–87

peristalsis Series of wave-like movements that propels food through the gut or digestive tract. It is caused by contractions of the smooth involuntary muscle of the gut wall. The reverse process, antiperistalsis, produces vomiting.

peritonitis Inflammation of the peritoneum – the strong connective tissue lining the abdominal walls and organs. It may be caused by bacterial infection or chemical irritation or it may arise spontaneously in certain diseases. Symptoms include fever, abdominal pain and distension and shock. Treatment is directed at the underlying cause.

phagocyte General name for LEUCOCYTES, including MACROPHAGES and neutrophils, able to engulf other cells, such as bacteria. Part of the body's IMMUNE SYSTEM, it digests what it engulfs in the defence of the body against infection. Phagocytes also act as scavengers by engulfing cells that die as part of the body's natural processes.

◀ *Phlebitis Coloured X-ray showing the inflammation of veins (known as phlebitis) in the leg of a patient. The veins (coloured orange) appear misshapen, leading off randomly (such as at left of image).*

lation. Two types of synthetic hormone, similar to OESTROGEN and PROGESTERONE, are generally used, though the former alone is effective in preventing ovulation; the latter helps to regulate the menstrual cycle. Possible side-effects include headache, HYPERTENSION, weight gain and a slightly increased risk of THROMBOSIS. *See also* CONTRACEPTION

pharmacology Study of the properties of DRUGS and their effects on the body.

pharmacopoeia Reference book listing drugs and other preparations in medical use. Included are details of their formulae, dosages, routes of administration, known side-effects and precautions.

phlebitis Inflammation of the wall of a vein. It may be caused by infection, trauma, underlying disease or the presence of VARICOSE VEINS. Symptoms include localized swelling and redness. Treatment includes rest and anticoagulant therapy.

physiology Branch of biology concerned with the functions of living organisms, as opposed to their structure (anatomy).

physiotherapy (physical therapy) Use of various physical techniques to treat disease or injury. Its techniques include massage, manipulation, exercise, heat, hydrotherapy, the use of ultrasonics and electrical stimulation.

pill, the Popular term for oral contraceptives based on the female reproductive HORMONES. They work by preventing ovu-

plague Acute infectious disease of humans and rodents caused by the bacillus *Yersinia pestis*. In humans, it occurs in three forms: **bubonic** plague, the most common and characterized by vomiting, fever and swellings of the lymph nodes called 'buboes'; **pneumonic** plague, in which the lungs are infected, and **septicaemic** plague, in which the bloodstream is invaded. Treatment is the administration of vaccines, bed rest, antibiotics and sulpha drugs. *See also* BLACK DEATH

plasma Straw-coloured, liquid part of BLOOD in which blood cells and PLATELETS are suspended. Plasma is 90% water with the remaining 10% made up of 100 solutes including plasma proteins, nutrients, carbon dioxide, nitrogenous wastes, hormones and ions.

plastic surgery Branch of surgery that involves the reconstruction of deformed, damaged or disfigured parts of the body. **Cosmetic surgery**, such as face-lifts, is performed solely to 'improve' appearance.

platelet Colourless, usually spherical structures found in mammalian BLOOD. Chemicals inside platelets, including calcium ions, enzymes and serotonin, are essential to the mechanism of blood clotting. The normal platelet count is *c.*300,000 per cu mm (0.000035 fl oz) of blood.

pleurisy Inflammation of the pleura – the membrane that lines the space between the lungs and the chest walls. It is nearly always due to infection, but may arise as a complication of other diseases.

pneumoconiosis Occupational disease of workers, principally miners, in confined and dusty conditions. Caused by inhaling irritants, often only as minute specks, the disease inflames and can finally destroy lung tissue.

pneumonia Inflammation of the lung tissue, most often caused by bacterial infection. Most at risk are the very young, the aged and those whose immune systems have been undermined by disease or certain medical treatments. The most common form is pneumococcal pneumonia, caused by the bacterium *Streptococcus pneumoniae*. Symptoms include fever, chest pain, coughing and the production of rust-coloured sputum. Treatment is with ANTIBIOTICS.

podiatry Treatment and care of the foot. Podiatrists treat such conditions as corns and bunions and devise ways to accommodate foot deformities.

poliomyelitis (polio) Acute viral infection of the nervous system affecting the nerves that activate muscles. Often a mild disease with effects limited to the throat and intestine, it is nonetheless potentially serious, with paralysis occurring in 1% of patients. It becomes life-threatening only if the breathing muscles are affected, in which case the person may need artificial ventilation. It has become rare in developed countries since the introduction of vaccination in the mid-1950s.

porphyria Group of rare genetic disorders in which there is defective METABOLISM of one or more porphyrins, the breakdown products of HAEMOGLOBIN. It can produce a wide range of effects, including intestinal upset, HYPERTENSION, weakness, abnormal skin reactions to sunlight and mental disturbance. A key diagnostic indicator is that the patient's urine turns reddish-brown if it is left to stand.

positron emission tomography (PET) Medical imaging technique (used particularly on the brain) that produces three-dimensional images. Radioisotopes, injected into the bloodstream prior to imaging, are taken up by tissues where they emit positrons that produce detectable photons. *See picture, p. 168*

post-mortem (autopsy) Dissection of a body to determine the cause of death. It

P

▶ *Poliomyelitis TEM of clusters of polio viruses, the cause of poliomyelitis. There are three serotypes of the polio virus. The serotype shown here is type 1, cause of most epidemics. Although rounded in shape (red) each virus has a cubic symmetry. They are picorna-viruses. RNA genetic material occurs in the core of each virus, surrounded by a protein coat (yellow). Infection occurs through the mouth. Usually only a mild illness results, but in more serious cases the virus may attack the nervous system causing paralysis or even death. Polio vaccines are available.*

P

is performed to confirm a diagnosis or to establish the cause of an unexpected death. **Morbid anatomy** (the examination of the dead) is a branch of PATHOLOGY.

post-natal depression Mood disorder, characterized by intense sadness, which may develop in a mother within a few days of childbirth. It ranges from mild cases of the 'baby blues', which are usually short-lived, to the severe depressive illness known as **puerperal psychosis**.

post-traumatic stress disorder Anxiety condition that may develop in people who have been involved in or witnessed some horrific event. It is commonly seen in survivors of battles or major disasters. The condition is characterized by repeated flashbacks to distressing events, hallucinations, nightmares, insomnia, edginess and depression. It usually recedes over time, but as many as 10% of sufferers are left with permanent psychological disability.

pregnancy Period of time from conception until birth, in humans normally c.40 weeks (280 days). It is generally divided into three periods of three months called trimesters. In the **first trimester**, the embryo grows from a small ball of cells to a fetus c.7.6 cm (3 in) in length. At the beginning of the **second trimester**, movements are first felt and the fetus grows to about 36 cm (14 in). In the **third**

trimester, the fetus attains its full body weight. *See also* LABOUR; Pregnancy and Childbirth, pp. 104–105

premature birth Birth of a baby prior to 37 weeks' gestation or weighing less than 2.5 kg (5.5 lb). Premature babies are more at risk than those born at full term and require special care.

prescription Order written by a doctor or dentist for drugs or other medication to be dispensed by a pharmacist. It should give details of the quantity of drugs to be dispensed, the dosage required, the route of administration (such as by mouth) and any precautions.

prickly heat Skin rash caused by blockage of the sweat glands in hot, humid weather. It occurs most often in infants and obese people. It disappears as the body cools.

progesterone Steroid hormone secreted mainly by the corpus luteum of the mammalian ovary and by the placenta during pregnancy. Its principal function is to prepare and maintain the inner lining (ENDOMETRIUM) of the uterus for pregnancy. Synthetic progesterone is one of the main components of the contraceptive PILL.

prolactin Hormone, secreted by the anterior pituitary gland, which stimulates the production of milk after childbirth. It also stimulates the secretion of proges-

◄ *Positron Emission Tomography (PET)* PET scans detect blood flow. These PET scans show areas of the brain activated by different tasks. At upper left, sight activates the visual area in the occipital cortex. Upper right, hearing activates the auditory area in the superior temporal cortex. Lower left, speaking activates the insula and motor cortex. Lower right, thinking about verbs and speaking them generates high activity in hearing, speaking, temporal and parietal areas.

P

▶ *Progesterone* Polarized light micrograph (PLM) of crystals of progesterone. Progesterone is the most potent of progestogens, a class of steroid hormones. It derives from pregnenolone. Its primary function is to prepare the inner lining of the womb for pregnancy. It is secreted by the ovaries after the release of an egg. If this egg is fertilized, the ovaries produce progesterone for four months, after which it is secreted by the placenta.

terone by the corpus luteum of the ovary. See also pp. 56–57 and 106–107

prolapse Displacement of an organ due to weakening of supporting tissues. It most often affects the rectum, due to bowel problems, or the uterus following repeated pregnancies.

prostaglandin Series of related fatty acids, with hormone-like action, present in SEMEN and liver, brain and other tissues. Their biological effects include the lowering of blood pressure and the stimulation of contraction in a variety of smooth muscle tissues, such as in the uterus.

prosthesis Artificial substitute for a missing organ or part of the body. Until the 17th century, artificial limbs were made of wood or metal, but innovations in metallurgy, plastics and engineering enabled lighter, jointed limbs to be made. More recent prosthetic devices include artificial heart valves made of silicone materials.

protein Organic compound containing many amino acids linked together by covalent, peptide bonds. Living cells use *c.*20 different amino acids, which are present in varying amounts. The GENETIC CODE is used to translate instructions in DNA that determine which amino acids are used and in which order they are combined. The most important proteins are enzymes, which determine all the chemical reactions in the cell, and antibodies, which combat infec-

tion. **Structural** proteins include KERATIN and COLLAGEN. **Gas transport** proteins include HAEMOGLOBIN. Nutrient proteins include casein. Protein HORMONES regulate the METABOLISM. See also ANTIBODY

Prozac Trade name for one of a small group of antidepressants, known as **selective serotonin re-uptake inhibitors** (SSRIs). They work by increasing levels of **serotonin** in the brain. Serotonin, or 5-hydroxytryptamine (5-HT), is a NEUROTRANSMITTER involved in a range of functions. Low levels of serotonin are associated with depression.

psittacosis (parrot fever) Disorder usually affecting the respiratory system of birds. Caused by a bacterium, it can be transmitted to human beings, producing pneumonia-like symptoms. Treatment is with ANTIBIOTICS.

psoriasis Chronic recurring skin disease featuring raised, red, scaly patches. The lesions frequently appear on the chest, knees, elbows and scalp. Treatment is with tar preparations, steroids and ultraviolet light. Psoriasis is sometimes linked with a form of ARTHRITIS.

psychosis Serious mental disorder in which the patient loses contact with reality, in contrast to NEUROSIS. It may feature extreme mood swings, delusions or hallucinations, distorted judgment and inappropriate emotional responses. **Organic** psychoses

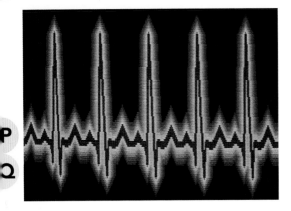

◀ *Pulse* Computer graphics abstract based on a section of the trace of a human pulse, the beat of the heart as it pumps blood around the body. Five successive beats are shown in this image.

may spring from brain damage, advanced SYPHILIS, senile DEMENTIA or advanced EPILEPSY. **Functional** psychoses, for which there is no known organic cause, include schizophrenia and MANIC DEPRESSION.

psychosomatic disorder Physical complaint thought to be rooted, at least in part, in psychological factors. The term has been applied to many complaints, including asthma, migraine, ulcers and hypertension.

puberty Time in human development when sexual maturity is reached. The reproductive organs take on their adult form and secondary sexual characteristics, such as the growth of pubic hair, start to become evident. Girls develop breasts and begin to menstruate; in boys there is deepening of the voice and the growth of facial hair. Puberty may begin at any time from about the age of ten, usually occurring earlier in girls than in boys. Hormones known as gonadotrophins regulated the process. *See also* pp. 108–109

pulse Regular wave of raised pressure in arteries that results from the flow of BLOOD pumped into them at each beat of the heart. The pulse is usually taken at the wrist, although it may be observed at any point where an artery runs close to the body surface. The average pulse rate is c.70 per minute in adults.

purpura Purplish patches on the skin due to seepage of blood from underlying vessels. Physical injury, vitamin deficiencies, some allergies and certain drugs are among the causes.

pus Yellowish fluid forming as a result of bacterial infection. It comprises blood serum, LEUCOCYTES, dead tissue, and living and dead BACTERIA. An ABSCESS is a pus-filled cavity.

pyelitis Inflammation of the renal pelvis, where urine collects before draining into the ureter. More common in women, it is usually caused by bacterial infection. Treatment is with ANTIBIOTICS and copious fluids.

quinine White, crystalline substance isolated in 1820 from the bark of the cinchona tree. It was once widely used in the treatment of MALARIA but has been largely replaced by drugs that are less toxic and more effective.

quinsy Inflammation of the tonsils, caused by an abscess, often a complication of TONSILLITIS. It is generally treated with ANTIBIOTICS.

rabies (hydrophobia) Viral disease of the central nervous system. It can occur in all warm-blooded animals, but is especially feared in dogs due to the risk of transmission to human beings. The incubation period varies from a week or two to more than a year. It is characterized by severe thirst, although attempting to drink causes painful spasms of the larynx. Other symptoms include fever, muscle spasms and delirium. Once the symptoms appear, death usually follows within a few days. Anyone bitten by a rabid animal may be saved by prompt injections of rabies vaccine and antiserum.

radiation sickness Illness resulting from exposure to sources of ionizing radiation, such as X-rays, gamma rays or nuclear fallout. Diarrhoea, vomiting, fever and haemorrhaging are symptoms. Severity depends upon the degree of radiation, and treatment is effective in mild cases.

radiology Medical speciality concerned with the use of radiation and radioactive materials in the diagnosis and treatment of disease. See also RADIOTHERAPY

▶ *Reflexology A chart indicating reflexology points on the foot. Areas of the foot thought to affect different parts of the body are coloured and numbered. Reflexology is a healing therapy originating from 'zone theory'.*

radiotherapy Use of radiation to treat TUMOURS or other pathological conditions. It may be done either by implanting a pellet of a radioactive source in the part to be treated, or by dosing the patient with a radioactive isotope or by exposing the patient to precisely focused beams of radiation from a machine such as an X-ray machine or a particle accelerator. Cobalt-60 is often used as it produces highly penetrating gamma radiation. In the treatment of CANCERS, the radiation slows down the proliferation of the cancerous cells.

reflex action Rapid involuntary response to a particular stimulus, e.g. the 'knee-jerk' reflex that occurs when the bent knee is tapped. It is controlled by the nervous system.

R

reflexology School of complementary medicine based on the theory that the image of the body is reflected in the foot. Modern practices are based on theories that date back as far as 3000 BC. Practitioners use foot massage to clear blockages of energy flow in the body, which cause illness.

repetitive strain injury (RSI) Pain and reduced mobility in a limb, most often the wrist, caused by constant repetition of the

◀ *Rickets* Coloured X-ray of the weakened bones and bowed legs of a child suffering from rickets. The skeleton of the legs appears deformed, with the long bones of the limbs severely curved. Rickets is caused by a nutritional deficiency of vitamin D. In adults, this condition is known as osteomalacia.

same movements. The symptoms arise from inflammation of the tendon sheaths because of excessive use. RSI is an occupational disorder mostly seen in assembly-line workers and keyboard operators.

respiration Series of chemical reactions by which complex molecules (food molecules) are broken down to release energy in living organisms. Enzymes control these reactions, which are an essential part of METABOLISM. There are two main types of respiration: aerobic and anaerobic. In **aerobic** respiration, oxygen combines with the breakdown products and is necessary for the reactions to take place. **Anaerobic** respiration takes place in the absence of oxygen. In most living organisms, the energy released by respiration is used to convert **adenosine diphosphate** (ADP) to **adenosine triphosphate** (ATP), which transports energy around the cell. At the site where the energy is needed, ATP converts back to ADP with the aid of a special enzyme and energy releases. The first stages of respiration take place in the cytoplasm and the later stages in the mitochondria. *See also* Respiratory system, pp. 74–79

resuscitation Measures taken to revive a person on the brink of death. The most successful technique available to the layman is **mouth-to-mouth** resuscitation. Medical staff receive instruction in **cardiopulmonary** resuscitation (CPR), which involves the use of specialized equipment and drugs to save patients whose breathing and/or heartbeat suddenly stop. *See also* FIRST AID

retrovirus Any of a large VIRUS family (Retroviridae) that, unlike other living organisms, contains the genetic material RNA (ribonucleic acid) rather than the customary DNA (deoxyribonucleic acid). In order to multiply, retroviruses make use of a special enzyme to convert their RNA into DNA, which then becomes integrated with the DNA in the cells of their hosts. Retroviruses include HIV, the virus that leads to AIDS (ACQUIRED IMMUNE DEFICIENCY SYNDROME).

rheumatic fever Inflammatory disorder characterized by fever and painful swelling of the joints. Rare in the developed world, it mostly affects children and young adults. An important complication is possible damage to the heart valves, leading to rheumatic heart disease in later life.

rheumatism A group of disorders with such symptoms as pain, inflammation and stiffness in the bones, joints and surrounding tissues. Usually ARTHRITIS is involved.

rhinitis Inflammation of the mucous membrane of the nose. It may be an allergic reaction (such as HAY FEVER) or a symptom of a viral infection such as the common cold.

rickets Disorder in which there is defective growth of bone in children: the bones fail to harden sufficiently and become bent. Due to either a lack of vitamin D in the diet or to insufficient sunlight to allow its synthesis in the skin, rickets results from the inability of the bones to calcify properly.

rigor mortis Stiffening of the body after death brought about by chemical changes in muscle tissue. Onset is gradual from minutes to hours. It disappears in c.24 hours.

ringworm Fungal infection of the skin, scalp or nails. The commonest type of ringworm is athlete's foot (*tinea pedis*). It is treated with antifungal preparations.

RNA (ribonucleic acid) Chemical (nucleic acid) that is involved in the synthesis of PROTEIN in a cell and is the genetic material in some viruses. Molecules of it in a cell are copied from DNA and consist of a single strand of nucleotides, each containing the sugar ribose, phosphoric acid and one of four bases: adenine, guanine, cytosine or uracil. **Messenger RNA (mRNA)** carries the information for protein synthesis from DNA in the cell nucleus to the ribosomes in the cytoplasm. **Transfer RNA** brings amino acids to their correct position on the mRNA. Each amino acid is specified by a sequence of three bases in mRNA.

roundworm Member of the invertebrate phylum Nematoda, a group of rounded, white worms with tapering ends, some of which are parasites in humans. Human infection with nematode larvae is through eating contaminated food, being bitten by infected blood-sucking insects or directly through cuts in the skin. Human nematodes include filarids (causing ELEPHANTIASIS) hookworms, pinworms and ascarids.

RSI Abbreviation of REPETITIVE STRAIN INJURY

rubella *See* GERMAN MEASLES

rupture *See* HERNIA

▶ *Salmonella Coloured TEM of* Salmonella *sp. bacteria. Each rod-shaped cell (blue/green) uses long hair-like flagellae (yellow) for motility.* Salmonella *bacteria are of the* Enterobacteriaceae *family. They are gram-negative bacilli that inhabit the gut. More than 1,800 different serotypes are known.*

saliva Fluid secreted into the mouth by the salivary glands. Human saliva consists of c.99% water with dissolved traces of sodium, potassium, calcium and the enzyme amylase. Saliva softens and lubricates food to aid swallowing and amylase starts the digestion of starches. *See also* pp. 84–85

salmonella Several species of rod-shaped BACTERIA that cause intestinal infections in human beings and animals. *Salmonella typhi* causes TYPHOID FEVER while other species cause GASTROENTERITIS. The bacteria are transmitted by carriers, particularly flies, and in food and water.

sarcoma Cancerous growth or TUMOUR arising from muscle, fat, bone, blood or

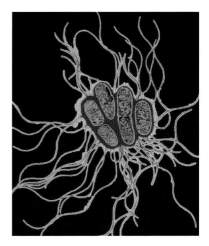

173

lymph vessels and connective tissue. *See also* CANCER

scabies Contagious infection caused by a female mite, *Sarcoptes scabiei*, which burrows into the skin to lay eggs. It can be seen as a dark wavy line on the skin and is treated with antiparasitic creams.

scanning In medicine, use of a non-invasive system to detect abnormalities of structure or function in the body. Detectable waves (X-rays, gamma rays or ultrasound) pass through the part of the body to be investigated and the computer-analysed results are displayed as images on a viewing screen.

scarlet fever (scarlatina) Acute infectious disease, usually affecting children, caused by BACTERIA in the *Streptococcus pyogenes* group. It is characterized by a bright red body rash, fever, vomiting and a sore throat. It is treated with ANTIBIOTICS.

schistosomiasis (bilharzia) Visceral, venous infestation of the human body by blood flukes of the genus *Schistosoma* occurring mainly in the tropics. Next to MALARIA, it is the most serious parasitic human infection. Symptoms are skin eruption, inflammation, fever and often swelling of the liver. It is contracted from water contaminated with microscopic larvae released by snail hosts.

The larvae enter the body through the skin, mature in the blood and deposit eggs throughout the body. Treatment is with drugs containing antimony or with a course of chemotherapy.

schizophrenia Severe mental disorder marked by disturbances of cognitive functioning, particularly thinking. As well as the characteristic loss of contact with reality, symptoms can include hallucinations and delusions and muffled or inappropriate emotions. Research suggests that schizophrenia may be caused by high levels of dopamine, a NEUROTRANSMITTER.

sciatica Severe pain in the back and radiating down one or other leg, along the course of the sciatic nerve. It is usually caused by inflammation of the sciatic nerve or by pressure on the spinal nerve roots.

sclerosis Degenerative hardening of tissue, usually due to scarring following inflammation or as a result of ageing. It can affect the brain and spinal cord, causing neurological symptoms, or the walls of the arteries.

screening In medicine, a test applied either to an individual or to groups of people who, though apparently healthy, are known to be at special risk of developing a particular disease. It is used to detect treatable diseases while they are still in the early stages.

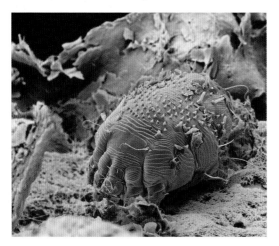

◀ *Scabies Coloured SEM of an itch mite,* Sarcoptes sp., *on the surface of a piece of skin. This parasite attacks human skin, causing scabies. Scabies is typified by severe itching (especially at night), red papules and often secondary infection. The female mite tunnels in the skin to lay her eggs and the newly hatched mites are passed easily from person to person by physical contact. The itching is caused by an allergic reaction to the mite's saliva or faeces. Magnification: ×110.*

► *Silicosis* False-colour X-ray of the chest area of a person suffering from silicosis, a lung disease caused by inhaling silica dust particles. The silica stimulates fibrosis of lung tissue (apparent as blue areas over both left and right lungs), which results in breathlessness and an increased susceptibility to tuberculosis. Workers in the mining, quarrying, stone-dressing, sandblasting and boiler-scaling industries are prone to the disease.

scurvy Disease caused by a deficiency of vitamin C (ascorbic acid), which is contained in fresh fruit and vegetables. It is characterized by weakness, painful joints and bleeding gums.

seasonal affective disorder (SAD) Mental depression apparently linked to the seasonally changing amount of light. Sufferers experience depression during autumn and winter.

seborrhoea Disorder of the sebaceous glands characterized by overproduction of sebum that results in red, scaly patches on the skin and dandruff.

sedative Drug used for its calming effect, to reduce anxiety and tension: at high doses it induces sleep. Sedatives include NARCOTICS, BARBITURATES and BENZODIAZEPINES.

semen Fluid in a male that contains sperm from the testes and the secretions of various accessory sexual glands. In men, each ejaculate is normally *c.*3 to 6 ml (1 to 2 fl oz) by volume, and contains *c.*200 to 300 million sperm. *See also* pp. 98–99

sepsis Destruction of body tissue by disease-causing (pathogenic) bacteria or their toxins. Local or widespread inflammation may occur, possibly followed by NECROSIS, the death of tissue. Treatment is with ANTIBIOTICS.

septicaemia Term for severe SEPSIS or BLOOD POISONING

serum Clear fluid that separates out if blood is left to clot. It is essentially of the same composition as PLASMA, but without fibrinogen and clotting factors.

sexual intercourse Term used to describe sexual relations between people. The term is most commonly used to describe the insertion of a man's penis into a woman's vagina. *See also* CONTRACEPTION; ORGASM; Reproductive system, pp. 98–103

sexually transmitted disease (STD) or sexually transmitted infection (STI) One of a number of infectious DISEASES that are spread from person to person by sexual contact, including vaginal and anal intercourse and oral sex, many of which are significant public health problems, especially among the young. STDs include gonorrhoea, SYPHILIS, HIV (the RETROVIRUS that causes ACQUIRED IMMUNE DEFICIENC SYNDROME or AIDS), CHLAMYDIA (which can cause pelvic inflammatory disease), genital HERPES and genital WARTS (which can trigger cervical CANCER in some women.

shingles (herpes zoster) Acute viral infection of sensory nerves. Groups of small blisters appear along the course of the affected nerves, and the condition can be very painful.

◀ *Smallpox Coloured TEM of a section through many Variola major viruses. These agents cause smallpox. The protein coat of each virus is coloured yellow and DNA red. The viruses display a complex symmetry. The disease causes high fever and skin spots that quickly develop into scarring pustules. The virus is transmitted by coughed droplets or the pus from pustules of an infected person. The virus is now used for purposes of biological research. Magnification: ×28,500.*

S

shock Acute circulatory failure, possibly with collapse. Caused by disease, injury or emotional trauma, it is characterized by weakness, pallor, sweating and a shallow, rapid pulse. In shock, blood pressure drops below the level needed to oxygenate the tissues.

Siamese (conjoined) twins Identical twins who are born physically joined together, sometimes with sharing of organs. Surgical separation is usually possible.

sickle-cell disease Inherited blood disorder featuring an abnormality of HAEMOGLOBIN. The haemoglobin is sensitive to a deficiency of oxygen and it distorts ERYTHROCYTES (red blood cells), causing them to become rigid and sickle shaped. Sickle cells are rapidly lost from the circulation, giving rise to anaemia and jaundice.

sight Sense by which form, colour, size, movement and distance of objects are perceived. Essentially, it is the detection of light by the eye, enabling the formation of visual images. *See also* pp. 50–53

silicosis Chronic lung disease, caused by prolonged inhalation of silica dust in occupations such as mining and stone grinding. *See picture*, p. 175

sleep Periodic state of unconsciousness from which a person or animal can be roused. During an ordinary night's sleep, there are intervals of deep sleep associated with rapid eye movement (REM) sleep. It is during this REM sleep that dreaming occurs. Studies have shown that people who are deprived of sleep become grossly disturbed. Sleep requirement falls sharply in old age. Difficulty in sleeping is called INSOMNIA. *See also* DREAM

sleeping sickness Popular name of two diseases. **Trypanosomiasis** is a disease of tropical Africa caused by a parasite transmitted by the tsetse fly. It is characterized by fever, headache, joint pains and anaemia. Ultimately, it may affect the brain and spinal cord, leading to profound lethargy and sometimes death. **Encephalitis lethargica** is a rare viral disease of the brain characterized by headache and drowsiness progressing to coma. It occurs in epidemic and sporadic forms and, most notoriously, was the cause of an epidemic that followed World War I, leaving many helpless survivors.

slipped disc (prolapsed intervertebral disc) Protrusion of the soft, inner core of an intervertebral disc through its covering, causing pressure on the spinal nerve roots. It is caused by a sudden mechanical force on the spine. It causes stiffness and

SCIATICA. Initial treatment is with strong painkillers. Physiotherapy is often used.

smallpox Formerly a highly contagious viral disease characterized by fever, vomiting and skin eruptions. It remained endemic in many countries until the World Health Organization (WHO) campaign, launched in the late 1960s. Global eradication was achieved by the early 1980s. As late as the 18th century, smallpox killed one in ten children born in France.

smell (olfaction) Sense that responds to airborne molecules. The **olfactory receptors** in the nose can detect even a few molecules per million parts of air. *See also* Taste and smell, pp. 48–49

snakebite Injection of potentially lethal snake venom into the bloodstream. There are three types of venomous snake: the **Viperidae**, subdivided into true vipers and pit vipers, whose venom causes internal haemorrhage; the **Elapidae** (including cobras, mambas and kraits), whose venom paralyzes the nervous system and the **Hydrophidae**, Pacific sea snakes with venom that disables the muscles. Treatment for all three types is with anti-venoms.

sodium bicarbonate (sodium hydrogen carbonate, $NaHCO_3$, popularly known as bicarbonate of soda) White, crystalline salt that decomposes in acid or on heating to release carbon dioxide gas. It has a slightly alkaline reaction and is an ingredient of indigestion medicines.

spasm Sustained involuntary muscle contraction. It may occur in response to pain or as part of a generalized condition, such as spastic paralysis or TETANUS.

sphygmomanometer Instrument used to measure BLOOD PRESSURE. The instrument incorporates an inflatable rubber cuff connected to a column of mercury with a graduated scale. The cuff wraps around the upper arm and inflates to apply tension to a major artery. When the air slowly releases, blood pressure readings can be ascertained from the scale.

spina bifida Congenital disorder in which the bones of the spine do not develop properly to enclose the spinal cord. Surgery to close the defect is usually performed soon after birth, but this may not cure disabilities caused by spina bifida. Taking folic acid in early pregnancy reduces the risk.

▶ *Staphylococcus Coloured SEM of Staphylococcus aureus bacteria (yellow) on human nasal epithelial cells. These gram-positive cocci (spherical bacteria) are adhering to mucus (blue) on the hair-like cilia which protrude from the epithelial cells. S. aureus is very common in humans, living harmlessly on the skin and in the nose, throat and large intestine. However it can multiply inside blocked skin pores, causing pus to build up and forming an acne spot or boil. Inside the body this bacteria may cause abscesses and suppurative infection. Magnification: ×7,000.*

spinal tap (lumbar puncture) Procedure for withdrawing CEREBROSPINAL FLUID from the lumbar (lower back) portion of the spinal cord for laboratory examination to aid diagnosis.

sprain Injury to one or more ligaments of a joint caused by sudden overstretching. Symptoms include pain, stiffness, bruising and swelling. Treatment includes resting and supporting the affected part before gentle mobilization.

squint *See* STRABISMUS

staphylococcus Spherical bacterium found in grape-like clusters on the skin and mucous membranes of humans. Pathogenic staphylococci cause a range of local or generalized infections, including PNEUMONIA and SEPTICAEMIA. They may be destroyed by ANTIBIOTICS, although some strains, notably the 'superbug' MRSA (methicillin-resistant *Staphylococcus aureus*) have become resistant. *See picture*, p. 177

sterility Inability to reproduce. It may be due to INFERTILITY or, in humans and other animals, to STERILIZATION.

sterilization Surgical intervention that terminates the ability of a human or other animal to reproduce. In women, the usual procedure is tubal ligation: sealing or tying off the fallopian tubes so that fertilization can no longer take place. In men, a VASECTOMY is performed to block the release of sperm. The term is also applied to the practice of destroying microorganisms in order to prevent the spread of infection. Techniques include heat treatment, irradiation and the use of disinfecting agents. *See also* pp. 98–103

steroid Class of organic compounds with a basic molecular structure of 17 carbon atoms arranged in four rings. Steroids are widely distributed in animals and plants, the most abundant being the sterols, such as CHOLESTEROL. Another important group are the steroid hormones, including the corticosteroids, secreted by the adrenal cortex, and the sex hormones (OESTROGEN,

PROGESTERONE and TESTOSTERONE). Synthetic steroids are widely used in medicine. Athletes sometimes abuse steroids to increase their muscle mass, strength and stamina, but there are harmful side-effects. Taking steroids is illegal in sports.

stethoscope Instrument that enables an examiner to listen to the action of various parts of the body, principally the heart and lungs. It consists of two earpieces attached to flexible rubber tubes that lead to either a disc or a cone.

stimulant Substance that increases mental alertness and activity. There are a number of stimulants that act on the central nervous system, notably drugs in the AMPHETAMINE group. Many common beverages, including tea and coffee, contain small quantities of the stimulant caffeine.

strabismus (squint) Condition in which the eyes do not look in the same direction. It may result from either disease of or damage to the eye muscles or their nerve supply, or an error of refraction within the eye.

streptococcus Genus of gram-positive spherical or oval BACTERIA that grow in pairs or bead-like chains. They live mainly as PARASITES in the mouth, respiratory tract and intestine. Some are harmless but others are pathogenic, causing SCARLET FEVER and other infections. Treatment is with ANTIBIOTICS.

stroke (apoplexy) Interruption of the flow of blood to the brain. It is caused by blockage or rupture of an artery and may produce a range of effects from mild impairment to death. Conditions that predispose to stroke include ARTERIOSCLEROSIS and HYPERTENSION. Many major strokes are prevented by treatment of risk factors, including surgery and the use of anticoagulant drugs. **Transient ischaemic attacks** (TIAs), or 'mini-strokes', which last less than 24 hours, are investigated to try to prevent the occurrence of a more damaging stroke.

strychnine Poisonous alkaloid obtained from the plant *Strychnos nux-vomica*. In the past, it was believed to have therapeutic value in small doses as a tonic. Strychnine poisoning causes symptoms similar to those of TETANUS, with death occurring due to SPASM of the breathing muscles.

sudden infant death syndrome (SIDS) (Cot death) Unexpected death of an apparently healthy baby, usually during sleep. The peak period seems to be around two months' old, although it can occur up to a year or more after birth. Claiming more boys than girls, it is more common in winter. The cause is unknown, but a number of risk factors have been identified, including prematurity and respiratory infection.

sulphonamide drug Any of a group of DRUGS derived from sulphanilamide, a red textile dye, that prevents the growth of bacteria. Introduced in the 1930s, sulphonamides were the first antibacterial drugs, prescribed to treat a range of infections. They were replaced by less toxic and more effective ANTIBIOTICS.

sunburn Damage to skin caused by prolonged or unaccustomed exposure to sunlight. It varies in severity from redness and soreness to the formation of large blisters. Excessive exposure to sunlight is

associated with the skin CANCER known as **melanoma**.

sunstroke Potentially fatal condition caused by overexposure to direct sunlight, in which the body temperature rises to 40.5°C (105°F) or more. Symptoms include hot, dry skin, exhaustion, vomiting, delirium and coma. Urgent medical treatment is required, possibly in an intensive care unit. Recovery is usual within a day or two.

surgery Branch of medical practice concerned with treatment by operation. Traditionally, it has mainly involved open surgery: gaining access to the operative site by way of an incision. However, the practice of using ENDOSCOPES enabled the development of 'keyhole surgery', using minimally invasive techniques. Surgeons perform operations under sterile conditions using local or general ANAESTHESIA.

syncope See FAINTING

synovial fluid Viscous, colourless fluid that lubricates the movable joints between bones. It is secreted by the synovial membrane. Synovial fluid is also found in the **bursae**, membranous sacs that help to reduce friction in major joints.

S

▶ *Stroke A 'stroke' is a disruption of the blood supply to the brain and is due either to a haemorrhage from a cerebral blood vessel (**A**), a thrombus (**B**) or an embolus (**C**). The damage (stippled area) may be permanent, but the outcome of a stroke depends on the extent and area of the brain affected by it. The symptons can range from a temporary loss of speech or other brain function and paralysis of the limbs to sudden death. A stroke on one side of the brain affects the limbs of the opposite side of the body because of the crossing over of nerve tracts in the brain stem (**D**). There is a similar effect on the visual cortex (**E**). Normal vision (**1**) is impaired on the left side (**2**) by a stroke on the right side.*

T

syphilis SEXUALLY TRANSMITTED DISEASE caused by the spiral-shaped bacterium (spirochete) *Treponema pallidum*. Untreated, it runs its course in three stages. The first symptom is often a hard, painless sore on the genitals, appearing usually within a month of infection. Months later, the second stage features a skin rash and fever. The third stage, often many years later, brings the formation of growths and serious involvement of the heart, brain and spinal cord, leading eventually to blindness, insanity and death. The disease is treated with ANTIBIOTICS.

tachycardia Increase in heart rate beyond the normal. It may occur after exertion or because of excitement or illness, particularly during fever, or it may result from a heart condition.

tapeworm Parasite of the genus *Taenia*, which colonizes the intestines of vertebrates, including human beings. Caught from eating raw or undercooked meat, it may cause serious disease.

tears Salty fluid, secreted by glands, that moistens the surface of the eye. It cleanses and disinfects the surface of the eye and also brings nutrients to the cornea.

temperature In biology, intensity of heat. In warm-blooded (endothermic) animals, body temperature is maintained within narrow limits regardless of the temperature of the surroundings. This is accomplished by muscular activity, the operation of cooling mechanisms, such as vasodilation, vasoconstriction and sweating and by metabolic activity. In humans, normal body temperature is *c*.37°C (98.6°F), but this varies with the degree of activity. In cold-blooded (poikilothermic) animals, body temperature varies more widely, depending on the temperature of the surroundings.

testosterone STEROID hormone secreted mainly by the mammalian testes. It is responsible for the growth and development of male sex organs and male secondary sexual characteristics, such as voice change and facial hair.

tetanus (lockjaw) Life-threatening disease caused by the toxin secreted by the anaerobic bacterium *Clostridium tetani*. The symptoms are muscular spasms and rigidity of the jaw, which then spreads to other parts of the body, culminating in convulsions and death. The disease is treated with anti-tetanus toxin and ANTIBIOTICS.

◀ *Testosterone* Polarized light micrograph (PLM) of testosterone crystals. Testosterone may be used in hormone replacement therapy to treat delayed puberty in boys, hypogonadism and some types of impotence. In women, it may be effective in the treatment of breast cancer.

► *Tetanus* False-colour SEM of Clostridium tetani, *the species of gram-positive, spore-forming, rod-like bacteria that causes tetanus. The spherical endospore appears as a swelling on top end of each bacterium. One resting endospore is produced from one vegetative bacterial cell and germinates to give rise to a single cell (i.e. the process is not one of multiplication). C. tetani exists harmlessly in the intestines of humans but becomes pathogenic (causes tetanus) when introduced through a wound. Magnification: ×4,700.*

T

tetracyclines One of a group of broad-spectrum ANTIBIOTICS that are effective against a wide range of bacterial infections.

thalassemia (Cooley's anaemia) Group of hereditary disorders characterized by abnormal bone marrow and erythrocytes (red blood cells). The predominant symptom is ANAEMIA, requiring frequent blood transfusions.

thalidomide Drug originally developed as a mild hypnotic, but whose use by women in early pregnancy until the early 1960s came to be associated with serious birth deformities. It is still manufactured for occasional use in the treatment of LEPROSY and ACQUIRED IMMUNE DEFICIENCY SYNDROME (AIDS).

thrombophlebitis Inflammation of the walls of veins associated with THROMBOSIS. It can occur in a woman's legs during pregnancy.

thrombosis Formation of a blood clot in an artery or vein. Besides causing loss of

circulation to the area supplied by the blocked vessel, thrombosis carries the risk of EMBOLISM.

thrush (candidiasis) Fungal infection of the mucous membranes, usually of the mouth but also sometimes of the vagina. Caused by the fungus Candida albicans, it is sometimes seen in people taking broad-spectrum ANTIBIOTICS.

thyroxine Hormone secreted by the thyroid gland. It contains iodine and helps regulate the rate of metabolism; it is essential for normal growth and development. *See also* pp. 56–59

tic Sudden and rapidly repeated muscular contraction, limited to one part of the body, especially the face.

tomography Technique of X-RAY photography in which details of only a single slice or plane of body tissue are shown.

tonsillitis Acute or chronic inflammation of the tonsils caused by bacterial or viral

T

◀ *Tuberculosis* Coloured chest X-ray of the lungs of a patient suffering from tuberculosis of the lung. The upper lobe of the lung (red, at left) is affected showing opacities (green). Healthy lung fields are black and the heart is at centre. Tuberculosis is a disease in which the lungs develop dense opacities marking the infected sites. The infection is passed from person to person in airborne droplets. Symptoms include coughing, fever, chest pain and shortness of breath. It is diagnosed by chest X-ray and sputum tests and is treated with antibiotic drugs.

infection. It is signalled by fever, a sore throat and difficulty in swallowing. Chronic tonsillitis is often treated by surgical removal of the tonsils (tonsillectomy).

toxicology Study of poisonous substances and their effects on living things.

toxic shock syndrome Potentially fatal condition in which there is a dangerous drop in blood pressure and rapid onset of fever, diarrhoea, vomiting and muscular pains. It is caused by BLOOD POISONING (septicaemia) arising from toxins put out by bacteria that normally reside in the body without causing harm. The syndrome is most often seen in young women using tampons during menstruation.

toxin Poisonous substance produced by a living organism. The unpleasant symptoms of many bacterial diseases are due to the release of toxins into the body by BACTERIA. Many moulds, some larger fungi and seeds of some higher plants produce toxins. The venom of many snakes contains powerful toxins. *See also* SNAKEBITE

toxoplasmosis Disease caused by the protist *Toxoplasma gondii*, which is transmitted from animals to human beings. It produces symptoms that are generally mild and flu-like in adults, but it can damage the nervous system, eyes and internal organs.

trace elements Chemical elements that are essential to life but normally obtainable from the DIET only in small quantities. They are essential to the reactions of enzymes and hormones.

tracer, radioactive Radioactive substance that is introduced into the body so that its progress can be tracked by special diagnostic equipment. This technique may help in the diagnosis of conditions such as thyroid disease.

tracheotomy (tracheostomy) Surgical procedure in which an incision is made through the skin into the trachea to allow insertion of a tube to facilitate breathing. It is done either to bypass any disease or damage in the trachea or to safeguard the airway if a patient has to spend a long time on a mechanical ventilator. *See also* pp. 74–75

trachoma Chronic eye infection caused by the bacterium *Chlamydia trachomatis*, characterized by inflammation of the cornea with the formation of pus. A disease of dry, tropical regions, it is the major cause of blindness in the developing world.

tranquillizer Drugs prescribed to reduce anxiety or tension and generally for their calming effect. They are used to control the symptoms of severe mental disturbance, such as schizophrenia or manic depression. They are also prescribed to relieve depression. Prolonged use of tranquillizers can produce a range of unwanted side-effects.

transfusion, blood *See* BLOOD TRANSFUSION

transplant Surgical operation to introduce organ or tissue from one person (the donor) to another (the recipient); it may also refer to the transfer of tissues from one part of the body to another, as in grafting of skin or bone. Major transplants are performed to save the lives of patients facing death from end-stage organ disease. Organs routinely transplanted include the kidneys, heart, lungs, liver and pancreas. Experimental work continues on some other procedures, including small-bowel grafting. Many other tissues are commonly grafted, including heart valves, bone and bone marrow. The oldest transplant procedure is corneal grafting, which restores the sight of one or both eyes. In 1967, Christiaan Barnard performed the first successful heart transplant operation. Most transplant material is acquired from dead people, although kidneys, part of the liver, bone marrow and corneas may be taken from living donors.

trauma Any injury or physical damage caused by some external event such as an accident or assault. In psychiatry, the term is applied to an emotional shock or harrowing experience.

▶ *Tumour A tumour is a swelling composed of cells independent of the body's control mechanism, so they rapidly divide, invade and kill surrounding tissue. Cross-sections of a healthy (**A**) and a diseased liver (**B**) are shown. The tumour shows a loss of cellular and structural differentiation and is unlike the tissue of origin.*

tropical diseases Any of a number of diseases predominantly associated with tropical climates. Major ones are MALARIA, LEISHMANIASIS, SLEEPING SICKNESS, FILARIASIS and SCHISTOSOMIASIS (bilharzia). The infectious agents of tropical diseases include viruses, bacteria, protist, fungi and worms of various kinds. Many of these disease microbes are spread by insect vectors such as mosquitoes.

trypsin Digestive enzyme secreted by the pancreas. It is secreted in an inactive form that is converted into active trypsin by an enzyme in the small intestine. It breaks down peptide bonds on the amino acids lysine and arginine. *See also* pp. 88–89

tuberculosis (TB) Infectious disease caused by the bacillus *Mycobacterium tuberculosis.* It most often affects the lungs (pulmonary tuberculosis), but may involve the bones and joints, skin, lymph nodes, intestines and kidneys. One-third of the world's population is infected, and up to 5% of those infected eventually develop TB. Poor urban living conditions have lead to a resurgence of the disease in the United States and much of Europe, where previously it had been in decline. The BCG vaccine against TB was developed in the 1920s and streptomycin, the first effective treatment drug, became available in 1944. However, the bacillus shows increasing resistance to drugs and some strains are multi-resistant.

tumour Any uncontrolled, abnormal proliferation of cells, often leading to the formation of a lump. Tumours are classified as

T

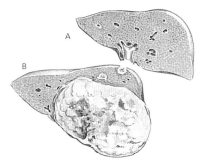

benign (non-cancerous) or malignant. *See also* CANCER

Turner's syndrome Hereditary condition in females, in which there is only one X-chromosome, instead of two. It results in short stature, infertility and developmental defects.

typhoid fever Acute, sometimes epidemic, communicable disease of the digestive system. Caused by *Salmonella typhi*, which is transmitted in contaminated water or food, it is characterized by bleeding from the bowel and enlargement of the spleen. Symptoms include fever, headache, constipation, sore throat, cough and skin rash.

typhus Any of a group of infectious diseases caused by rickettsiae (small bacteria) and spread by parasites of the human body such as lice, fleas, ticks and mites. **Epidemic** typhus, the result of infection by *Rickettsia prowazekii*, is the most serious manifestation. Associated with dirty, overcrowded conditions, it is mainly seen during times of war or famine.

ulcer Any persistent sore or lesion on the skin or on a mucous membrane, often associated with inflammation. Ulcers may be caused by infection, chemical irritation or mechanical pressure.

urethritis Inflammation of the urethra. It is usually due to a SEXUALLY TRANSMITTED DISEASE (STD) but may also arise from infection.

urine Fluid filtered out from the bloodstream by the KIDNEY. It consists mainly of water, salts and waste products such as urea. From the kidneys it passes through the ureters to the bladder for voiding by way of the urethra. *See also* pp. 96–97

urology Medical speciality concerned with the diagnosis and treatment of diseases of the urinary tract in women and of the urinary and reproductive systems in men.

urticaria *See* HIVES

vaccination Injection of a VACCINE in order to produce IMMUNITY against a disease. In many countries, children are routinely vaccinated against infectious diseases.

vaccine Agent used to give IMMUNITY against various diseases without producing symptoms. A vaccine consists of modified disease organisms, such as live, weakened virus or dead ones that are still able to induce the production of specific antibodies within the blood. *See also* ANTIBODY; IMMUNE SYSTEM; VIRUS

Valium Proprietary name for diazepam, a sedative drug in the BENZODIAZEPINE group. It is used in the treatment of anxiety, muscle spasms and epilepsy.

varicose vein Condition where a vein becomes swollen and distorted. Varicose veins can occur anywhere in the body, but are commonly found in the legs.

vasectomy Operation to induce male sterility, in which the tube (*vas deferens*) carrying sperm from the testes to the penis is cut. A vasectomy is a form of permanent CONTRACEPTION, although in some cases the operation is reversible.

vasoconstrictor Any substance that causes constriction of blood vessels and, therefore, decreases blood flow. Examples include NORADRENALINE, angiotensin and the hormone vasopressin (also known as antidiuretic hormone, or ADH).

vasodilator Substance that causes widening of the blood vessels, permitting freer flow of blood. Vasodilator drugs are mostly used to treat HYPERTENSION and ANGINA.

venereal disease (VD) Derived from 'Venus', the Roman goddess of love, term used until the 1990s, but now obsolete, to describe SEXUALLY TRANSMITTED DISEASES especially GONORRHOEA and SYPHILIS, two diseases that can be treated with antibiotics, as can CHLAMYDIA, the commonest sexually transmitted disease reported today. Genital HER-PES and HIV infections, both viral, are incurable but their effects can be lessened by drugs. All these diseases are usually transmitted through contact between the mucous membrane of the penis and that of the vagina or rectum.

verruca In medicine, form of WART on the sole of the foot, which is painful because it is forced to grow inwards. Like other warts, it is due to infection with the human papillomavirus.

vertigo Dizziness, often accompanied by nausea. Due to disruption of the sense of balance, it may be produced by ear disorder, reduced flow of blood to the brain caused by altitude, emotional upset or spinning rapidly.

virology Study of VIRUSES. The existence of viruses was established (1892) by D Ivanovski, a Russian botanist, who found that the causative agent of tobacco mosaic disease could pass through a

▶ *Virus Bacteriophages are viruses that infect bacteria. Bacteriophage lambda (A) is a virus that infects E. coli bacteria in the intestine. The DNA (1) is stored in a polyhedral protein head (2) attached to a hollow tail (3) with a single tail fibre (4). The phage attaches itself to a bacterium (B) at the tail (1) and injects its DNA (2). This can result in an infection that causes the cell to lyse (break open), releasing replica phages. During such an infection, the phage DNA remains separate from the bacterial DNA (3) and uses the cell's enzymes to synthesize the proteins that make up the new phages (4). The phage DNA replicates (5). In the process, the bacterial DNA is used and, by the time the cell lyses (6), it may be destroyed. The injection of phage DNA may result in a lysogenic infection (7), when the phage DNA becomes part of the bacterial chromosome (8). Cell division (9) then produces numerous replicas of the phage DNA. During the course of the lysogenic growth, damage to the cell may result in a lytic infection (10) by causing the phage DNA to be ejected from the bacterial chromosome.*

porcelain filter impermeable to BACTERIA. The introduction of the electron microscope in the 1940s made it possible to view viruses. *See also* VIRUS

virus Infectious chemical package. Viruses vary in size from 10 to 300 nanometres, and contain only genetic material in the form of DNA or RNA. Viruses are incapable of independent existence: they can multiply only when they enter another cell, such as a bacterium or animal cell because they lack energy-releasing and protein-synthesizing functions. When they enter a cell, viruses subvert the host's metabolism so that viral reproduction is favoured. Control of viruses is difficult because harsh measures are required to kill them. The animal body has, however, evolved some protective measures, such as production of INTERFERON and of antibodies directed against specific viruses. Where the specific agent can be isolated, VACCINES can be developed, but some viruses change so rapidly that vaccines become ineffective. *See artwork,* p. 185. *See also* ANTIBODY; IMMUNE SYSTEM

vomiting Act of bringing up the contents of the stomach by way of the mouth. Vomiting is a reflex mechanism that may be activated by any of a number of stimuli, including dizziness, pain, gastric irritation or SHOCK. It may also be a symptom of serious disease.

W

wart Raised and well-defined small growth on the outermost surface of the skin, caused by the human papillomavirus. It is usually painless unless in a pressure area, as with a VERRUCA.

whooping cough (pertussis) Acute, highly contagious childhood respiratory disease. It is caused by the bacterium *Bordetella pertussis* and is marked by spasms of coughing, followed by a long-drawn intake of air, or 'whoop'. It is frequently associated with vomiting and severe nose bleeds. Immunization reduces the number and severity of attacks.

World Health Organization (WHO) Intergovernmental organization, a specialized agency of the United Nations (UN). Founded in 1948, it collects and

◀ *X-ray* False-colour anteroposterior X-ray of a normal adult, female pelvis. The pelvis is formed by the sacrum, coccyx and two innominate (hip) bones. Here, the sacrum is at top centre, articulating with each innominate bone at the sacroiliac joints. Left and right hip bones meet at the pubic symphysis (bottom). Also visible is the articulation of the rounded head of each femur (thigh bone) with each hip socket.

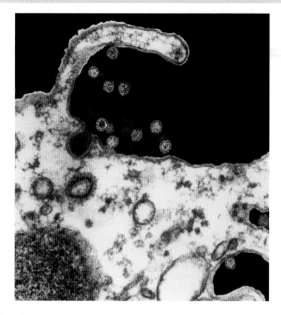

► **Yellow fever** *Coloured TEM of yellow fever viruses (yellow/red, at centre) on the surface of an infected cell. The cell is white/brown. This virus occurs in tropical Africa and Central and South America. It is transmitted to humans when an infected female mosquito* Aedes aegypti *bites a human. Yellow fever is so-called because it may cause yellowing of the skin due to jaundice. About 10% of victims die. Magnification: ×50,000.*

shares medical and scientific information and promotes the establishment of international standards for drugs and vaccines. The WHO has made major contributions to the prevention of diseases such as malaria, polio, leprosy and tuberculosis, and the eradication of smallpox. Its headquarters are in Geneva in Switzerland.

X-ray Electromagnetic radiation of shorter wavelength (or higher frequency) than visible light, produced when a beam of electrons hits a solid target. Wilhelm Röntgen discovered X-rays in 1895. They are normally produced for scientific use in X-ray tubes. Because they are able to penetrate matter that is opaque to light, X-rays are used to investigate inaccessible areas, especially of the body.

yaws (framboesia) Contagious skin disease found in the humid tropics. It is caused by a spirochete (*Treponema pertenue*), related to the organism causing SYPHILIS. Yaws is not a SEXUALLY TRANSMITTED DISEASE (STD), but rather is transmitted by flies and by direct skin contact with the sores. It may go on to cause disfiguring bone lesions.

yellow fever Acute infectious disease marked by sudden onset of headaches, fever, muscle and joint pain, jaundice and vomiting: the kidneys and heart may also be affected. It is caused by a VIRUS transmitted by mosquitoes in tropical and subtropical regions. It may be prevented by vaccination.

zoonosis Any infection or infestation of animals that is transmissible to human beings.

187

Index

Page numbers in *italic* type refer to illustrations or their captions; **bold** numbers refer to major references.

collarbone *see* clavicle
colon 10, 91
colostrum 107
colour blindness 52, **53**
columnar tissue 11
compact tissue 16–17, *16*
complement 72
conception 102, *102*, 104
concha 75
cone 50, 51, 52–3, *52*
congenital malformation 104
conjunctiva *50*
connective tissue 10, 11, 30
consciousness 36, 37, 38
contractions, uterine 106, 107
convoluted tubule *94*, 95
cornea 50, *50*, 52, *52*
corpus albicans *100*
corpus callosum 36, *36*
corpus cavernosa 99, *99*, 102
corpus luteum *100*, 101, *101*, 103
corpus spongiosum 99, *99*, 102
cortical tissue 16–17, *16*
corticosteroid 57
costal cartilage *14*, 21
coughing 38, 80, **81**
coxal bone *14*, **24–5**
cranial bones 18–19, *18*, *19*
cranial cavity 5, 18
cranial nerve **43**, *49*
cranium 18
crawling 108
creativity 36, 37
cricoid cartilage 80, *80*, *81*
cross bridge 33
crossing over 111, *111*
cuboidal tissue 11
cutaneous membrane 11
cytoplasm 6, *6*
cytosine 8, *9*

D

defecation 91
deltoid *28*
dementia 109
dendrite 35, *35*
dentine 85, *85*, 108
deoxyribonucleic acid (DNA) 8–9, *8*, *9*, 91, 110, 111
bases 8, *9*
depression 31
dermatome *41*
dermis 11, 12, *12*, 13, *47*
descending tract 40
detoxification 92, 93
diapedesis 65
diaphragm 4, *10*, *47*, 76, 78–9, *78*, 81
diencephalon 36, 37
diffusion 6
digestion 34, 82, 90
chemical 82
mechanical 82
digestive juices *10*, 11
digestive system 5, *10*, 11, 44, **82–95**
parasympathetic nervous system 45
diploid cells 8

disaccharide 83, 84
disease 11, 12
dominant allele 110–11
Down's syndrome 111
ductus arteriosus 63
duodenum 86, *86*, 87, 88–9, *88*, 90, *93*
dura mater (meninge) *40*, 41

E

ear 11, 14, 37, 46, **54–5**
and balance 38, 54, **55**
embryo 104
external auditory meatus 18, *18*
see also hearing
eardrum 54, 55
ectoderm 103, *103*
egestion 82
egg *see* ovum
ejaculation 45, 98, 99, 102
elastic cartilage 11
elastin 11, 12
elbow *26*, 30, *31*
electrons 7
elevation 31
embryo 101, 102, **103–5**, 111
emotion 34, 36, 37, **39**
enamel, tooth 85, 108
endocardium 63
endocrine system 11, 34, 37, **56–9**
endoderm 103, *103*
endolymph 54
endometrium 101, *101*, 102, 103, 104
endoplasmic reticulum (ER)
rough 6, *7*
smooth 7
endothelium 68, *68*
energy 74, 82
chemical 32
heat 32
kinetic 32
enterokinase 91
enzyme 8, 44–5, 82, 87, 89, **90–1**
eosinophil 66, *66*
epidermis 10, 12, *12*, 13, *47*
epididymis 98, *98*, 99, *99*
epiglottis *10*, 11, *48*, 74, 75, 80, *80*, 84, 85
epimysium 32, *32*
epineurium *42*
epithelia *see* epithelial tissue
epithelial tissue 10–11, *10*, 90
erection 44, 98, 100, 102, 108
ergometrine 107
erythrocyte *see* red blood cell
erythropoiesis 66
erythropoietin 66
ethmoid bone 18, *18*
eustachian tube 54
exhalation **78–9**
exocrine cell 89
extension, muscular 30, 31
extensor reticulum *28*
external oblique *28*
extremities *see* limbs

eye 34, 37, 38, 46, **50–3**
colour 51, *111*
embryo 104
focus 50, 52, *52*, 108
movement 38, *43*
pupil reflex 44, 45, **50–1**
see also vision
eyeball **50**
eyebrow 13
eyelash 13, 50
eyelid 50, 104
eye socket *see* orbit

F

face 19
facial bones 18, *18*, 19, *19*
facial expression 18, *43*
facial hair 13, 99
facial nerve 43
faeces 82, 91, 95
fallopian tube 10, 100, *100*, *101*, 102
fascicle 32, 42, *43*
fat (dietary) 82, 83, 87, 89, 90, 91
fat storage 11, 15, 17
fatty acid 83, 90, *90*, 91
feet 104
female 4–5, *4*, *24*, **100–1**
femur *14*, 17, 24, 25, *25*
fertilization 8, 101, **102**, 111
fetus 102, 104, **105–7**
circulation 63
skull 19
fever 72
fibre, dietary 82
fibre, tissue 11
fibrin 67, *67*
fibrous cartilage 11
fibula *14*, 15, 25, *25*, 27
fight or flight response 38, 57
fimbria 100, *100*, *101*
finger 13, *13*, *22*, *23*, 47, 104
fixator 30, 31
flexion, muscular 30, 31
flexor carpi radialis *28*
follicle 101
see also Graafian follicle
follicle-stimulating hormone (FSH) 58, 59, 98, 101
follicular cyst *100*
fontanelle 19, *19*
food 82
see also digestive system
foot 4, **25**, *26*, 30
foramen 18
intervertebral *42*
vertebral *21*
foramen magnum 18, 40
forearm 4, *4*, 22–3, *23*
forebrain 36–7
forehead 18
foreskin 99
fornix 36, 37, *39*
fovea 50, 51, 53
fracture 17
frontal bone 18, *19*
frontalis *28*
frontal lobe 36, *36*, *39*
fulcrum 30
fundus 86, *86*

G

gall bladder *10*, 82, 88, **89**, 90, *93*
gamete 98, 100, **110–11**
ganglion 40, *42*, 45
gas exchange **76–7**
gastric juice 72, 75, 86–7
gastrin 86
gastrocenemis *28*
genes 9, **110–11**
dominant 110–11
recessive 111
genetic abnormality 111
genome 9, 110
gland *see* endocrine system
glans 99
glenoid cavity 22, *23*
glia 11, 34_5
glial cells *see* glia
glomerulus 94–5, *94*
glossopharyngeal nerve *43*
glottis 80–1, *80*
glucagon 57, 89, *89*, 93
glucose 8, 32, 44–5, 57, 74, 83, 89, 90, 91, **92–3**, 94
gluteus maximus *28*
glycerol 90
glycolysis 7
glycoproteins 6
golgi complex 6, *7*
goose pimples 13
Graafian follicle *100*, 101, *101*
granulocyte 65, 66
grey matter 37, 38, 40, *40*
ground substance 11
growth 82, **108**
bones 17
growth hormone (GH) 11, 58, 59
guanine 8, *9*
gyrus 36

H

haematoma *17*
haemoconcentration 37
haemocytoblast 66
haemoglobin 65, 67, 89, 95, 107
haemolysis 67, 107
hair 12, **13**, *47*
colour 13, 109
erector muscles 12, *13*
follicles 12, *12*, 13
lanugo 105
loss 13, 109
old age 109
hamate bone *22*
hand 4, **22–3**
embryo 104
haploid cells 8
hard palate 19, *49*, 74, 84, *84*
haustrum 91
Haversian canal *16*
head 4, 18–19, *18*, *19*
movement 18, 30
hearing 46, **54–5**
heart 4, *5*, *10*, *47*, **60–3**, 64, 74
embryo 104
see also cardiac muscle
heartbeat 63, 102
fetal 105